THE MEDITERRANEAN DIET
COOKBOOK FOR TWO

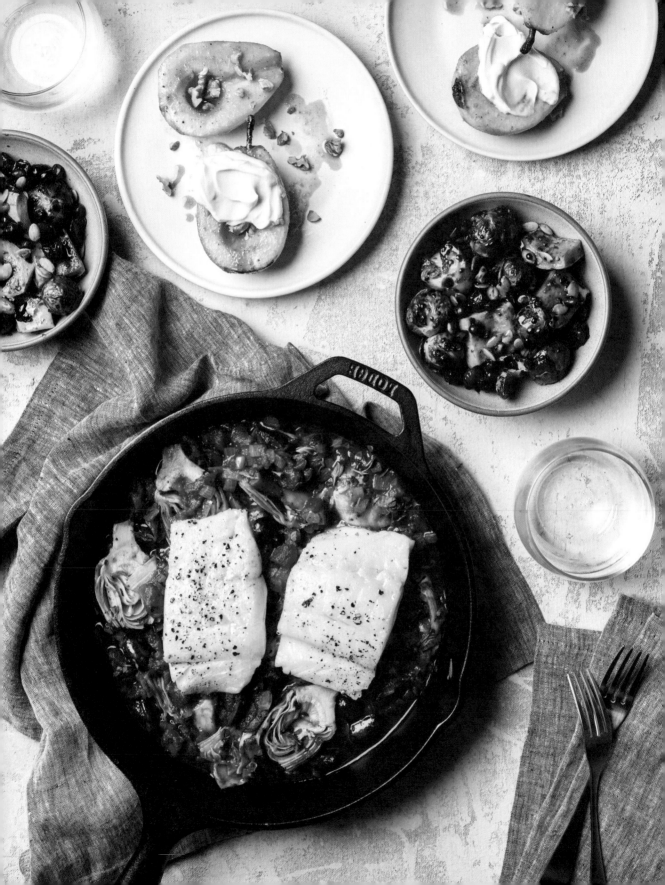

THE MEDITERRANEAN DIET COOKBOOK FOR TWO

100 Perfectly Portioned Recipes for Healthy Eating

Anne Danahy, RDN

Photography by Thomas J. Story

CALLISTO PUBLISHING

Published by Callisto Publishing LLC C/O Sourcebooks LLC
P.O. Box 4410, Naperville, Illinois 60567-4410
(630) 961-3900
callistopublishing.com

Printed and bound in China.
OGP 14

To my family and friends, who are always more than happy to eat; to Cait and Ryan, my favorite taste testers and kitchen companions; to Bob, for encouraging me to do hard things; to Mom and Dad, for always making family dinners a priority.

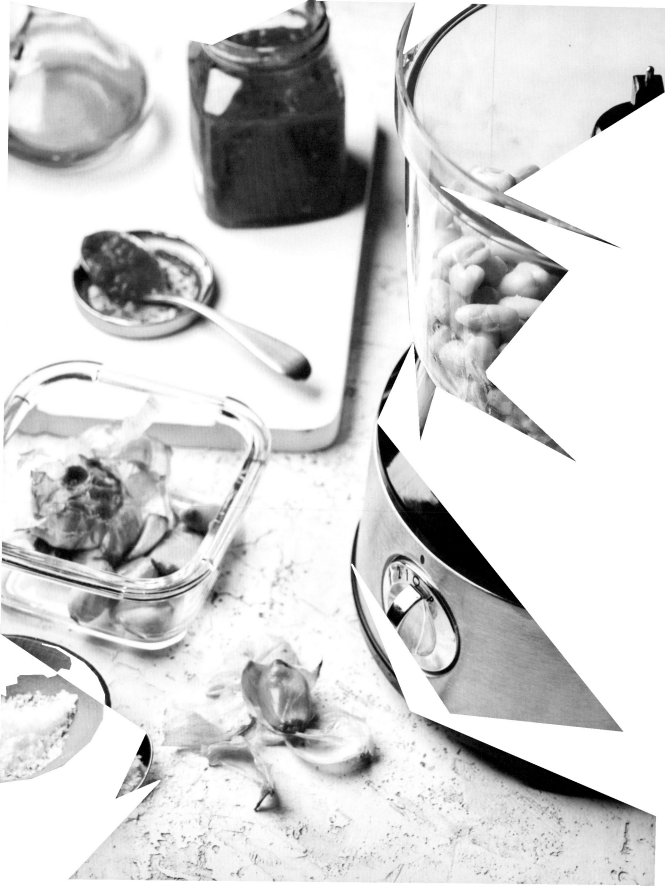

CONTENTS

Chapter 7: Fish and Seafood Mains   93

Chapter 8: Poultry Mains   111

Chapter 9: Beef, Pork, and Lamb Mains 131

Chapter 10: Simple Sides 147

Chapter 11: Desserts and Sweets 163

INTRODUCTION

No matter how skilled of a cook you are, there's something extremely satisfying about preparing a meal from good, wholesome ingredients, and sharing it with family, a friend, or your partner.

Cooking draws people together, sparks conversation, and, importantly, it's one of the easiest things you can do with others to create a healthier lifestyle. However, I also appreciate that cooking requires time for preparation, as well as planning and shopping. When you're cooking for two, it might not seem worth the effort—but trust me, it's time very well spent.

As a registered dietitian, the most satisfying part of my job is inspiring people to get into the kitchen and discover just how delicious healthy meals can be. It's my favorite part of working with clients, and the reason I've been sharing recipes and tips on my nutrition blog, *Craving Something Healthy*, for the past six years. I'm absolutely thrilled when someone reports back about the health benefits they've experienced from cooking and eating better.

My family and I have always loved to cook and experiment in the kitchen, and over the years we've moved more toward the Mediterranean diet. It's partly because of the research on its health benefits, which include lower rates of heart disease, diabetes, cancer, and depression. We also like our food to taste great too, and that's the main reason we've gone Mediterranean.

We've been extremely fortunate to visit several Mediterranean countries as a family, and the food was always a highlight. The way cooks use fresh ingredients like lemons, oranges, and herbs to elevate simple dishes of grilled whole fish and platters of fresh vegetables has inspired me to appreciate the flavors of fresh, seasonal food.

Whether you're just learning to cook, you're an empty nester in need of some new, scaled-back recipes, or your health-care provider has recommended incorporating the Mediterranean diet into your lifestyle, it's my hope that *The Mediterranean Diet Cookbook for Two* will inspire you to spend some quality time in the kitchen discovering some new, delicious, and healthy recipes.

This book is full of the kinds of meals I prepare in my own kitchen. I love all foods, but much like the traditional Mediterranean diet, I lean more toward vegetarian and seafood-based meals because they're fresh, light, and quick and easy to prepare. Thus, you'll find quite a few recipes based around vegetables, fruits, legumes, whole grains, yogurt, and seafood. They're staples in my kitchen, and I've highlighted their specific health benefits as well as given lots of tips and shortcuts throughout that may be helpful. Because I also believe all foods can fit into a healthy diet, you'll also find an assortment of "special occasion foods" or those to eat in moderation, like meats and even desserts.

As an empty nester, I understand how frustrating it is when most recipes make far more portions than needed. Therefore, except for soups and stews—which I love for leftovers—I've made it a priority to scale these recipes down to just two portions to minimize food waste and encourage more variety. I've also included specific sizes on canned goods, weights for proteins, and staples to stock, so you can buy only what you need and not have half-used ingredients living in the back of your refrigerator.

In addition to discovering new, healthy recipes for two from this book, I also hope you'll be inspired to work with a partner to incorporate the other aspects of the Mediterranean diet: adding in more physical activity, making meals more social, and taking time to enjoy the small pleasures in life. As you'll learn, all of these things work together to promote a happier, healthier, and more fulfilling life. Having someone along for the journey not only makes it more fun, but also increases the chances of success for both of you!

In good health,
Anne Danahy

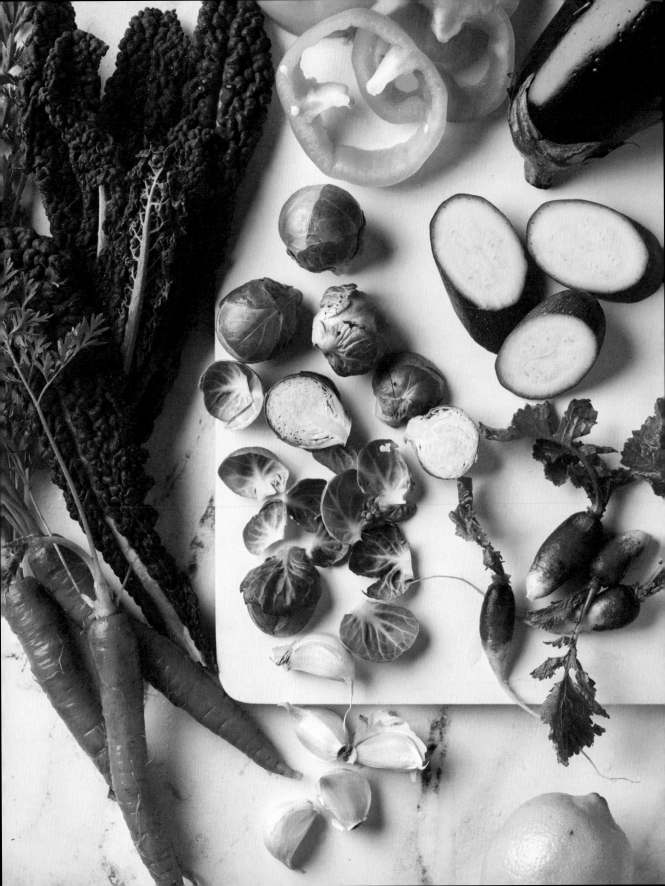

CHAPTER 1

OVERVIEW OF THE MEDITERRANEAN DIET

The countries and cultures in the Mediterranean region have long adhered to a simple way of eating that's based on whole foods, primarily plants, seafood, and healthy fats. When these foods are enjoyed in balanced amounts, they have tremendous health benefits for both your body and mind. It's a simple concept that's being backed by more and more scientific research.

I've long enjoyed the foods and flavors of the Mediterranean diet, not only because of how they taste, but also because of the way they make me feel. This chapter will introduce you to the Mediterranean diet, including the basic principles of the diet, as well as the foods most commonly eaten and their health benefits. You'll also find information and tips for incorporating the Mediterranean lifestyle into your own.

WHAT IS THE MEDITERRANEAN DIET?

Unlike other diets that emphasize counting calories and avoiding certain foods, the Mediterranean diet is about enjoying more fresh ingredients and meals that are prepared from scratch as much as possible. It's about slowing down to eat, enjoying meals with friends and family, and incorporating more joyful movement into your daily life.

There's a very good reason this diet is ranked among one of the best year after year, and why it's so often recommended by medical professionals. Rather than a structured diet plan, the Mediterranean diet is a diet pattern—an overall style of eating and living that's lifelong, rather than short-term. It's also a delicious way to reduce your risk of chronic diseases like heart disease, diabetes, cancer, and even Alzheimer's disease.

Research suggests that the specific foods, eating patterns, and lifestyle in the Mediterranean region all contribute to better health and longer lives. In fact, the Mediterranean diet is associated with improved cholesterol, blood sugar, blood pressure, and weight, and it has advantages for brain and neurological health.

Meals that fit the Mediterranean diet are rich in fruits, vegetables, whole grains, seafood, and healthy fats such as nuts, seeds, and olive oil. This diet pattern also includes smaller portions of fermented dairy, eggs, poultry, and even an occasional glass of wine with your meals.

More than 20 countries are part of the Mediterranean region. It includes European countries, such as Spain, France, Italy, Greece, Turkey, and Croatia. It also covers parts of northern Africa, including Morocco, Tunisia, and Egypt, and the Middle East, including Syria and Israel. If your family has roots in any of these countries, the Mediterranean diet is already in your blood!

One of the most attractive things about the Mediterranean diet is its flexibility, incorporating ingredients from any of these countries. Plus, flavor profiles from other parts of the world can easily be tailored to a "Mediterranean" style of eating. As long as a dish is made from whole food ingredients and is rich in plants and healthy fats, it can work as part of a Mediterranean diet pattern.

Just as important as the food is the lifestyle as a whole, which is the definition of wellness. People who live in this region get more daily physical activity—whether it's walking to the store or working in the garden. They're socially connected, with a strong sense of community. They also make it a point to take time out for meals and eat at a slower pace. These simple acts all contribute to better overall health.

8 Principles of the Mediterranean Diet

The diet is focused on the same core food groups you already know, but more than likely they're prepared and served in a different way. *How* they are eaten—more slowly, mindfully, and with family and friends—is just as important as what is eaten. The diet is based around the following eight simple principles:

1. **Focus on vegetables.** In each meal, fresh, colorful, seasonal vegetables are the stars of the plate. When you eat seasonally, you always enjoy freshness and variety.

2. **Change your thoughts around meat.** The Mediterranean diet calls for small amounts of poultry and meat, focusing instead on seafood and high-fiber legumes for protein. That doesn't mean meat is off-limits, but it's eaten in moderation, usually reserved for special occasions, and is always surrounded by vegetables.

3. **Let herbs and spices shine.** Whether they're dried or fresh, all herbs and spices add flavor, color, and tremendous health benefits to your meals.

4. **Embrace healthy fats.** Mediterranean is not synonymous with low fat. Instead, it features healthy, high-quality sources of fat. Olive oil is a staple ingredient in every kitchen, along with nuts, seeds, and olives.

5. **Enjoy quality dairy foods.** Unsweetened plain or Greek yogurt and cheese are traditional in the Mediterranean diet. However, like meat, they're eaten in smaller amounts and usually alongside fruits, vegetables, and other staple foods.

6. **Switch to ancient grains.** Instead of white or refined grains, which have been stripped of their nutrients, the Mediterranean diet features whole and cracked ancient grains like farro, barley, oats, and bulgur. Bread is a staple, but it's made with whole grains and is often a fermented sourdough.

7. **Highlight fruit as your dessert.** Fruits are full of natural sugars, and when served along with some nuts, a small portion of cheese, or baked into a dessert, they add fiber and nutrients while satisfying your sweet tooth.

8. **Make meals a celebration.** Mediterranean meals aren't about gourmet dining. They're about celebrating the simplicity of food and taking time to enjoy its fresh flavors with friends and family. Whenever possible, sit down at the table with someone you care about and take time to appreciate your meal and where it came from.

The Science Behind the Mediterranean Diet

Hundreds of research studies over the past 70 years indicate a wide range of health benefits for this way of eating. Here are a few landmark studies on the Mediterranean Diet:

THE SEVEN COUNTRIES STUDY

In 1947, Ancel Keys, a physiologist from Minnesota, was among the first to suggest that heart disease might be related to diet and lifestyle. He and other medical colleagues from around the world formally began the Seven Countries Study in the late 1950s to examine the relationship between diet, lifestyle, cholesterol levels, and heart disease risk among men in:

- Greece
- Southern Italy
- Croatia and Serbia (formerly Yugoslavia)
- Finland
- The Netherlands
- Japan
- The United States

This was one of the first studies to suggest that a diet rich in plant foods, along with more physical activity and less stress, was linked to lower heart disease. The men who seemed to have the lowest risk all lived in areas bordering the Mediterranean Sea.

THE LYON DIET HEART STUDY

Here, researchers in France found that people who had an initial heart attack had a lower risk of having a second one when they followed a Mediterranean diet versus a traditional Western-style low-fat diet. They found that the protective effect of the Mediterranean diet lasted for at least four years after following it.

THE NURSE'S STUDY

Researchers followed nearly 75,000 female nurses from 1984 to 2004 and found that those who ate a Mediterranean diet more often had a significantly lower risk of heart disease and stroke than those who followed it less often.

THE PREDIMED STUDY

This five-year study out of Spain showed that following a Mediterranean diet enriched with additional olive oil and nuts was linked with less death from cardiovascular disease and lower risk of developing diabetes.

GOOD FAT VS. BAD FAT

The effect of fat on our health has been debated for decades, and like so many other aspects of nutritional science, the recommendations have come full circle. For years, fat in general was thought to contribute to heart disease, but research has shown us that not all fat is created equal. Some types should be avoided, and others limited, but the fat that's prevalent in the Mediterranean diet is downright healthy.

The bad fats include hydrogenated fats, which should be completely avoided, and saturated fat, found in animal foods like meats and full-fat dairy, which should be limited. Although saturated fats can raise cholesterol levels, the jury is still out on their overall impact on health.

The good fats include monounsaturated and polyunsaturated fats found in olive oil, olives, nuts, seeds, and avocados. These help to reduce the inflammation in the body that contributes to heart disease, cancer, and other chronic diseases.

The Mediterranean Diet Food Pyramid

The Mediterranean diet food pyramid was designed by the Harvard School of Public Health, the World Health Organization, and Oldways Preservation Trust, a food and nutrition nonprofit. It's a visual guideline that makes the principles of the diet easy to understand and follow.

Vegetables, fruits, whole grains, olive oil, legumes, nuts, seeds, herbs, and spices make up the base or the widest part of the pyramid, because these are foods to eat at every meal.

Seafood, especially oily fish, occupies the next level and should be eaten often, or at least twice each week. Poultry, eggs, cheese, and yogurt follow, with a guideline of eating moderate portions daily to weekly.

The smallest part of the pyramid represents meat and sweets, which should be enjoyed less often and reserved for special occasions.

Water is the beverage of choice. However, if you enjoy red wine, it does have some heart health benefits when consumed in moderation—although it may not be appropriate for everyone.

Health Benefits

Fad diets come and go because they're hard to stick to, and their effects are usually short-lived. The Mediterranean diet, however, is here to stay. It's not only tasty and satisfying, but also easy to follow for life. In addition, it's backed by significant research on heart disease and a wide range of other benefits.

REDUCES THE RISK OF HEART DISEASE

Study after study over the decades confirms that the Mediterranean diet reduces the overall risk of death from cardiovascular disease, especially heart attack and stroke. The diet pattern works by improving cholesterol levels, reducing plaque buildup in the arteries, and contributing to stronger, less stiff, and healthier blood vessels.

BENEFICIAL FOR WEIGHT MANAGEMENT

Although there is no emphasis on calories, even from fat, planning your meals and snacks around the Mediterranean style of eating can still result in weight loss, especially abdominal fat, and an easier time maintaining a healthy weight.

THE MEDITERRANEAN DIET PYRAMID

As illustrated in the pyramid, fresh fruits and vegetables, grains such as whole-wheat bread, pasta, or rice, and olive oil are important parts of every meal. Foods enjoyed daily include nuts, cheese, or yogurt, and red wine. Fish, eggs, poultry, and legumes are consumed several times a week, and meat is restricted to a few times a month.

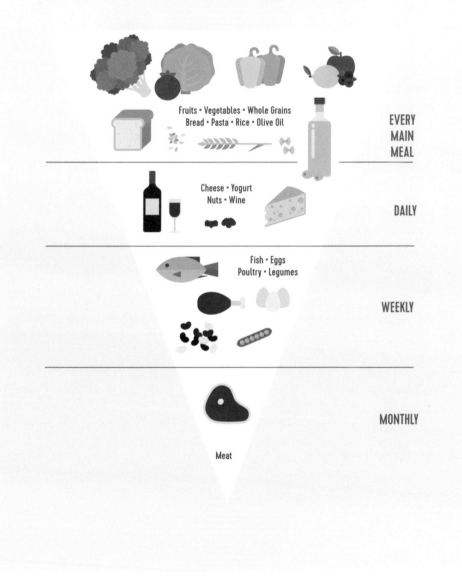

MAY REVERSE METABOLIC SYNDROME

Metabolic syndrome is a cluster of symptoms that includes high blood pressure, high blood sugar or insulin resistance, high triglycerides, low HDL ("good") cholesterol, and excess abdominal fat. Together, they increase your risk of diabetes and heart disease. People who eat a Mediterranean-style diet have a lower risk of developing metabolic syndrome, and what's more, switching to this diet pattern has even been shown to reverse it.

REDUCES THE RISK OF, AND HELPS MANAGE, DIABETES

If diabetes runs in your family, or if you have diabetes or prediabetes, following this healthy eating pattern has numerous benefits—and its emphasis on healthy fats is a big part of the reason. The diet itself has been shown to improve glucose levels, likely because it's low in added sugar and refined carbs. In addition, olive oil especially seems to help reduce the risk of diabetes.

IMPROVES BRAIN HEALTH AND COGNITIVE FUNCTION

Another area that researchers are examining is the diet's effects on brain health and cognitive function, not only with aging, but throughout the life cycle. For example:

- Eating the Mediterranean way during pregnancy can result in a healthier pregnancy and baby.

- Following the diet when you're in your twenties and thirties seems to result in less depression throughout adulthood.

- An Australian study found that in people who are at risk of developing Alzheimer's disease, or those who have early symptoms of it, the Mediterranean diet may slow the disease's progression.

MAY REDUCE THE RISK OF CANCER

The high antioxidant content of the Mediterranean diet can protect your cells and DNA from oxidative damage that triggers the growth of cancer cells. In particular, following a Mediterranean diet may reduce the risk of prostate, colorectal, breast, bladder, and endometrial cancers.

THE STANDARD AMERICAN DIET VS.
THE MEDITERRANEAN DIET

It's important to note that the Mediterranean diet is not just grabbing a handful of nuts for a snack or cooking with olive oil. It's definitely about the food, but it's also about the meal experience itself.

It starts with the quality of the food. The true benefits come from real, fresh, whole foods as opposed to packaged foods with a long list of ingredients. Many shortcut products, such as bottled salad dressings, packaged seasoning mixes, or jarred sauces, contain ingredients your body doesn't recognize, and they undermine your health.

It's also about how that food is eaten. While Americans often eat on the run, in a car, or alone, the Mediterranean diet is slow, thoughtful, consumed at the table, and, whenever possible, enjoyed with others. The sense of community has benefits that extend beyond the food.

The Importance of an Active Lifestyle

Although it's called a "diet," the Mediterranean diet is about more than just food. It's about a lifestyle. Interestingly, the word "diet" comes from the Greek word *diaita,* which means "way of living." Part of that way of living includes being physically active every day.

It's said that sitting is the new smoking. It causes weight gain and nearly doubles your risk of developing diabetes. It also increases your risk of cancer and heart disease. Moving more throughout the day, whether it's in the form of a gym workout or just incorporating more physical activity into your day, has tremendous benefits for both physical and mental health.

The Department of Health and Human Services has published guidelines on physical activity for Americans. They recommend all adults aim for at least 150 to 300 minutes of moderate intensity activity each week. Unless you're hitting the gym for at least an hour most days of the week, that's a lot more than most people do. If it sounds like a lot, start by making small changes in your routine—they'll all add up. Try some of the following tips. Once they become a habit, keep adding on to them week by week:

- Set a timer and get up every hour to stretch and walk for 5 minutes.

- Plan your errands so you can park centrally and walk from place to place.

- Park at the very back of the parking lot and walk the extra distance to work or the grocery store.

- Make it a priority to walk, jog, or bike for at least 45 minutes most days of the week.

- Plant a garden and tend to it yourself.

- Join a local walking or hiking group and get out on the weekends.

- Try to make physical activity a social event by taking classes or working out with friends. It helps you to stay motivated, and it's just more enjoyable.

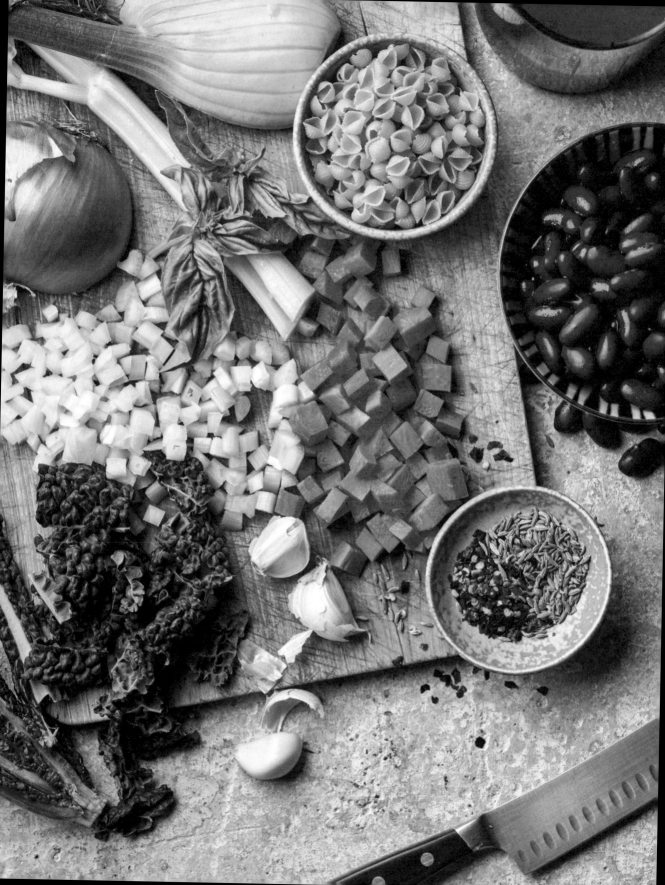

CHAPTER 2

MEDITERRANEAN COOKING FOR TWO

I'm an empty nester who loves to cook. Even though my kids have been out of the house for a while, I still find myself shopping in bulk and preparing more than we can eat sometimes. They're hard habits to break.

I've had to retrain myself to cook for two, but I'm finding that I enjoy better foods as a result. In addition, because the Mediterranean diet is focused on fresh flavor and simple preparations instead of complex cooking techniques, I actually spend less time in the kitchen.

In this chapter, you'll find helpful information about how to downsize your cooking. We'll cover things like how to shop, which foods to stock, where to save your money, and appropriate portion sizes when cooking for two.

MEDITERRANEAN PLATE PORTIONS

Unlike most other "diets" that require you to cut back, the Mediterranean diet isn't at all about deprivation. Instead, it's about *abbondanza*, which means plenty, or abundance, in Italian. However, Mediterranean plates look a little bit different than most American plates.

Foods eaten in abundance include vegetables, legumes, and seafood. They're high in nutrients but low in calories. Olive oil, nuts, and seeds help to keep you fuller and more satisfied, and they're consumed in smaller portions. There's a natural sense of balance to the diet, which minimizes the need for weighing, measuring, and calorie counting—and it's so refreshing!

When planning your meals, fill your plate, but keep these general guidelines in mind:

Start with ½ plate of vegetables. It doesn't matter if they're in the form of a salad, cooked, or raw, but they should fill at least half your plate. In the American diet, vegetables are considered a side dish, but in the Mediterranean diet, they're the star of the plate.

Satisfy your sweet tooth with fruit. Choose a 1-cup serving as dessert.

Fill about ⅓ of your plate with protein. Good choices to eat every day are legumes, dairy (milk, yogurt, or cheese), or seafood, the latter of which should be on your plate a minimum of twice each week. Choose poultry and eggs the rest of the time, but limit red meat to just a few times each month.

Keep your starch to a small portion. If desired, add one small serving—about ½ to 1 cup—of a cooked whole grain at each meal. I often recommend using your hand to measure a serving. If you could just about fill a scooped hand with cooked barley, oats, or any other grain, it's probably a good size portion for you.

Include a serving of healthy fat with each meal. Include about a tablespoon of olive oil, or a handful of nuts or seeds at each meal.

If you enjoy red wine, enjoy it in moderation. It's rich in antioxidants that are associated with heart health, but it should be limited to one 5-ounce glass per day for women and up to two glasses per day for men.

THE BALANCED PLATE

Being on a diet doesn't have to mean an empty plate. Go ahead—fill your plate!

But before you start scooping, picture how you will fill your plate. A balanced plate—one that provides the right ratio of foods—looks like this:

Good protein sources include poultry, fish, and lean meat that are grilled, baked, or broiled.

Some starches include peas, corn, beans, pasta, bread, alcohol, potato, sweet potato, butternut squash, and quinoa and other whole grains.

Be extra mindful of portions of what I call "calorically dense" foods: avocado, oils, nuts, and nut butters. Even though these contain healthy fats and are good for us, they're high in calories. Reasonable portion sizes would be one-fourth of an avocado, 1 tablespoon nut butter or oil, and 10 to 15 nuts.

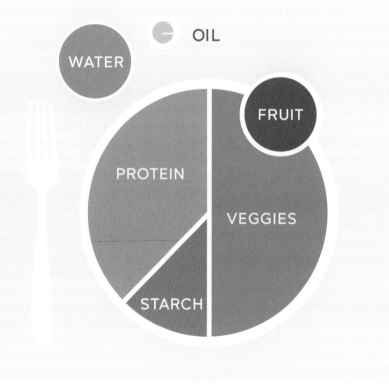

THE MEDITERRANEAN PANTRY

Eating the Mediterranean way means planning your meals and snacks around the following categories of foods on a very regular basis. These are the foods that will become a familiar part of your diet and, as such, should fill your grocery cart each week.

Vegetables and fruits. Although it's not a vegetarian diet, vegetables and fruits make up the bulk of meals and snacks on the Mediterranean diet. They're all sources of important nutrients and antioxidants that prevent chronic diseases. They also provide an average of 5 grams of fiber per serving, which helps meet your daily fiber goal of at least 25 grams per day as recommended by the FDA. When you consider that a serving of vegetables has only about 25 calories, and a serving of fruit has about 60 calories, it's easy to see how they help balance your plate in the Mediterranean diet.

Legumes. These include dried beans and peas like cannellini beans, chickpeas (garbanzo beans), lentils, kidney and black beans, split peas, and many other types. They're high in protein, low in fat and sodium, and a source of many nutrients. Importantly, they're also a source of soluble fiber, the kind that lowers your cholesterol, stabilizes your blood sugar, and helps keep you full. Eating about a ½-cup serving most days is linked with a healthier weight and lower risk of heart disease, diabetes, and many types of cancer.

Fish and seafood. Fatty fish like salmon, sardines, anchovies, and mackerel are the best sources of omega-3 fats. These healthy fats provide tremendous anti-inflammatory benefits for both your body and brain. Other whitefish or shellfish are lower in these fats, but are still full of essential vitamins, minerals, and lean protein. They're great choices to include in your meal plan, because eating any kind of fish is linked with a lower risk of cardiovascular disease. The Mediterranean diet favors fish over other meats or poultry; it's a staple source of protein that can be eaten as often as you like.

Olive oil. Nothing else is as much a part of the Mediterranean diet as olive oil. Olive trees are some of the oldest cultivated trees in the Mediterranean region. Olives are technically a fruit, but they're quite high in fat—most of which is monounsaturated and can lower your cholesterol. Using olive oil as part of the Mediterranean diet has been shown to not only promote healthier cholesterol levels, but also reduce the risk of heart disease, diabetes, and metabolic syndrome.

Nuts and seeds. These are also important sources of healthy fat, as well as some protein. Because they're high in fat and calories (and let's face it, they're expensive too), the best way to eat all nuts and seeds is by incorporating them into meals and snacks.

Fermented dairy foods. Dairy gets a bad rap sometimes, but it's actually an important source of protein in the Mediterranean diet. I'm not talking about chocolate milk or ice cream here! Instead, unsweetened fermented milk products like yogurt and kefir, along with high-quality Parmesan and cheeses made from sheep, goat, or water buffalo milk are the best choices. Fermented dairy foods are naturally low in sugar, easier to digest, and are an important source of gut-friendly probiotics.

Foods to Stock

When your kitchen is well stocked, there's no excuse to not eat well! Base most meals around these and have them readily available:

Produce: Any fresh, seasonal, and local is best, if available, but frozen fruits without sugar and plain frozen vegetables are great backups.

Legumes: Cannellini, kidney, black beans, lentils, split peas, chickpeas, or any other dried or canned beans.

Nuts and seeds: Almonds, walnuts, pecans, pistachios, chia, hemp, sunflower, pumpkin, and sesame seeds. Only buy what you'll use within a few months and store them in airtight jars.

Herbs and spices: Any fresh or dried.

Olive oil: It degrades quickly once it's opened, so only buy as much as you'll use within two months, and store it in a cool, dark pantry or cabinet—not in the sun or next to the stove.

Whole or cracked grains: Oats, brown or wild rice, quinoa, farro, freekeh, barley, bulgur, sorghum, and millet are all nutritious grains.

Fish and seafood: Salmon, cod, haddock, halibut, flounder, wild shrimp, scallops, lobster, clams, mussels, canned or fresh sardines, mackerel, anchovies, light tuna (white tuna is higher in mercury so eat it less frequently).

Foods to Moderate

In general, animal-based foods should be eaten less frequently on the Mediterranean diet. They're higher in saturated fat and although they are a good source of protein, they don't have the disease-preventing antioxidants and fiber that plant foods provide. Try to eat small to moderate portions of these foods daily or several times weekly.

Dairy: Plain, unsweetened Greek or regular yogurt or kefir; an assortment of cheeses such as Parmesan or Romano, goat, or ricotta; cow's milk if desired.

Eggs: FYI—the only difference between brown and white eggs is the color of the hens that lay them!

Poultry: Choose skinless chicken breast or thighs.

Foods to Limit

The following foods are linked to higher risk of heart disease, cancer, and obesity, and they may promote inflammation, which contributes to more chronic disease. They should all be eaten in moderation and used more for flavor than as a big part of your meal.

Red meat: Beef, bison, veal, pork, lamb, goat, and prosciutto should be eaten in moderation, so save these for special occasions, and eat small 3- or 4-ounce portions. Meats processed with nitrates are linked to cancer and should be avoided. These include cured sausages, hot dogs, bacon, salami, pepperoni, and many cold cuts. For a healthier option, look for items labeled "nitrate-free."

Butter, lard, margarine: These are all saturated fats that raise cholesterol levels and contribute to heart disease. Use them sparingly.

Sugar: Sweets and desserts that are high in processed sugars (not natural fruit sugar) add calories, increase inflammation and abdominal fat, and contribute to heart disease, diabetes, metabolic syndrome, and even some types of cancer. Choose fruit, or fruit-based desserts that are lightly or naturally sweetened, and save sugary desserts for an occasional treat.

DECODING PACKAGED FOOD LABELS

You're not alone if you find food labels confusing! To simplify them, first look at the calories, to make sure they seem reasonable. If a food costs you a large portion of your daily calorie allowance, put it down.

Next, check to see if there's added sugar. There are many different names for sugar: agave nectar, barley malt syrup, brown rice syrup, corn syrup, dextrose, and fructose are some. It's important to limit as much added sugar as possible because it adds extra calories and is linked to obesity and increased risk of diabetes.

Finally, glance through the ingredients list. Highly processed foods have a long list of ingredients, and most of them don't come from nature. These foods cause abdominal weight gain and promote inflammation in your body. If a food contains a lengthy and unrecognizable list of ingredients, choose something else.

Some commonly used food additives that you should pass on include:

- artificial colors (e.g., red 20, blue 1, yellow 6)
- artificial flavors
- artificial sweeteners (e.g., acesulfame K, aspartame, sucralose)
- preservatives (e.g., BHT, nitrate/nitrate, polysorbate-60, potassium bromate)

A helpful resource to learn more about food additives and their safety profiles is the Center for Science in the Public Interest's Chemical Cuisine, at https://cspinet.org/eating-healthy/chemical-cuisine.

Ideally, look for foods that are minimally processed and include just three or four familiar ingredients. And keep in mind, the healthiest foods (fruits and vegetables) don't require a food label!

SHOPPING FOR TWO

It sounds so easy. However, if you're just starting out and not used to cooking at all, or if you're an empty nester who has been cooking for a family for years, shopping and cooking for two can be a challenge. To make matters worse, food often comes in larger packages, and most cookbooks and recipes are created to make four to eight servings. Unless you're prepared to eat the same thing day after day, or freeze part of the recipe, there's lots of waste.

To make shopping and cooking for two as easy as possible, I've scaled everything down here. With the exception of just a few recipes—most of which are soups, which I think make sense to make in larger quantities and eat more than once—I've designed these recipes to make just two portions. That said, most of them can also be scaled up if you want to make it once and eat it a few times.

Here are some tips that I've found helpful when transitioning from grocery shopping for a family, to shopping for two:

Plan your meals for the week. Write out your meals and keep a grocery list on your phone so you'll have it at the store.

Maximize your prep time. Do a little extra work tonight and save time tomorrow. If a recipe calls for half an onion, chop the entire thing and save half for tomorrow; instead of preparing just one cup of a whole grain, make several and use them throughout the week.

Go for quality over quantity. Since you're buying less food, treat yourself to better quality and invest in your health.

Pay attention to food waste. If you're finding that you're wasting more food by shopping in bulk, drop your membership club or use it only for items you really use a lot of. It's probably a better idea to shop for smaller amounts of fresh produce twice a week, and buy just the amount of fish, poultry, or meat you need at the fish or meat counter. Stock up on things like bulk grains, nuts, and olive oil a few times a year because they have a much longer shelf life.

SERVING SIZES FOR COMMON FOODS

It can be helpful—and eye-opening—to be aware of the portions you eat. Here are some serving size guidelines to follow:

EQUIVALENT		FOOD	CALORIES
Fist	¾ cup	Rice Pasta Potatoes	150 150 150
Palm	4 ounces	Lean meat Fish Poultry	160 160 160
Handful	1 ounce	Nuts Raisins	170 85
Thumb	1 ounce	Peanut butter Hard cheese	170 100

SAVING MONEY

There's a misconception that eating the Mediterranean way can break the bank. It's true that some healthier foods are more expensive, especially when you compare them to frozen dinners or fast-food dollar menu items. However, a healthier diet, a gym membership, and any other self-care expenses are really an investment in yourself.

Think of it this way: You can pay a little bit extra now to take care of yourself, or you can pay a lot more later in potential health care and medication expenses. If you reframe your thoughts about healthy foods, you can appreciate that you're worth the investment.

To save money and shop smarter, try these tips:

Purchase produce that's in season. It's frequently on sale, or lower priced.

Keep a stock of frozen fruits and vegetables on hand. As long as they don't contain sugar or sauces, they're every bit as healthy and they last for months.

Buy long-lasting items in bulk. Nuts, seeds, and whole grains will last for several months if you store them in airtight mason jars.

Take advantage of sale prices. Nonperishable items like canned beans and tomatoes are pantry must-haves. They're staples that are just as healthy as dried or fresh.

Substitute some canned fish instead of fresh. Some types, like mackerel or sardines are more readily available in cans or tins. They're nicely portion-controlled and a time-saver that still provides the health benefits of fresh fish. There are some high-quality brands out there, so try a few and find one you like.

Skip the high-end stores and brands. Today it's so easy to find good-quality, organic, and local products everywhere, from Walmart to your local grocery store to Whole Foods. Shop the store brands whenever possible.

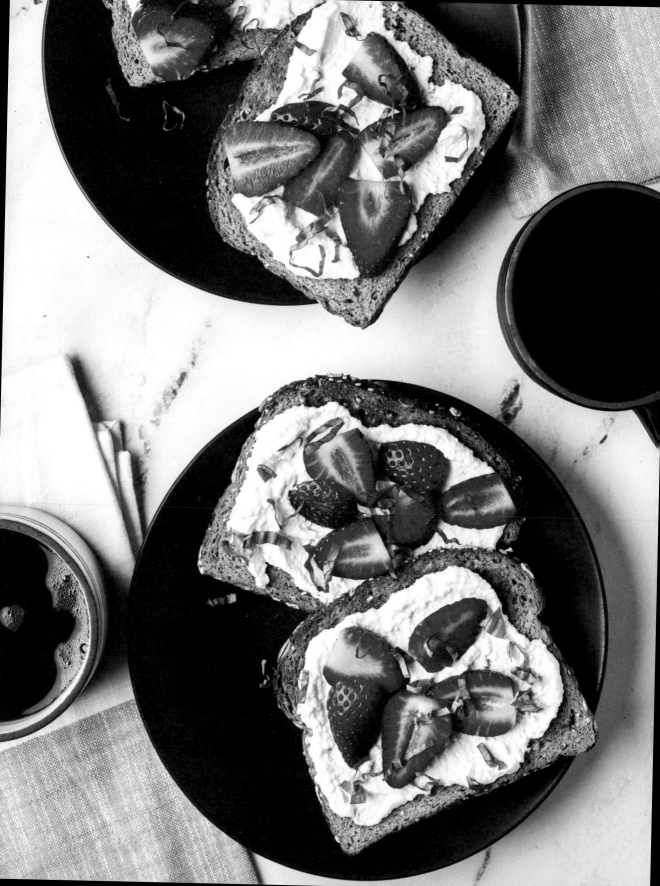

CHAPTER 3

BREAKFAST

Whether you wake up starving and ready to eat, or you prefer to ease your way into your first meal of the day, breakfast is your chance to start out the day on the right foot. Eating a satisfying meal that's full of fruits or vegetables, some whole grains, and protein gives your metabolism a jump start and often motivates you to make better choices throughout the rest of the day.

My basic rule for all meals and snacks, including breakfast, is to keep it balanced and include at least three different food groups on your plate or in your bowl.

< Strawberry Basil Honey Ricotta Toast, page 27

ORANGE CARDAMOM BUCKWHEAT PANCAKES

Prep Time: 15 minutes / Cook Time: 10 minutes / Serves 2
30 minutes, gluten-free, vegetarian

Buckwheat is an ancient grain that's naturally gluten-free. It's lower in carbs and higher in fiber, protein, vitamins, minerals, and antioxidants compared to regular wheat flour. Buckwheat not only boosts the nutrients in these pancakes but also gives them a rich, nutty flavor that's delicious with orange and cardamom. Serve these with a dollop of Greek yogurt, fresh orange slices, a sprinkle of pomegranate arils (seeds), and a drizzle of maple syrup if you like.

½ **cup buckwheat flour**

½ **teaspoon cardamom**

½ **teaspoon
baking powder**

¼ **teaspoon baking soda**

½ **cup milk**

¼ **cup plain Greek yogurt**

1 **egg**

½ **teaspoon
orange extract**

1 **tablespoon maple
syrup (optional)**

1. In a medium bowl, combine the buckwheat flour, cardamom, baking powder, and baking soda.

2. In another bowl, combine the milk, yogurt, egg, orange extract, and maple syrup (if using) and whisk well to combine.

3. Add the wet ingredients to the dry ingredients and stir until the batter is smooth.

4. Heat a nonstick skillet or a griddle over high heat. When the pan is hot, reduce the heat to medium.

5. Pour the batter into the pan to make four 6-inch pancakes. Depending on the size of your pan, you may need to do this in four batches.

PREP TIP: No matter how hard I try, my first pancake never works out! If that's you, don't waste a full-size pancake. Make a mini one using about a tablespoon of the batter and see if that one works. It's usually just a matter of getting the pan to the right temperature. Once you get it right, the rest will be fine.

Per Serving: Calories: 196; Total fat: 6g; Total carbs: 27g; Fiber: 3g; Sugar: 6g; Protein: 10g; Sodium: 242mg; Cholesterol: 93mg

STRAWBERRY BASIL HONEY RICOTTA TOAST

Prep Time: 10 minutes / Serves 2

30 minutes, vegetarian

Ricotta cheese is often overlooked unless you're making lasagna for a crowd. However, it's a great source of protein and full of calcium. It's also a nice, silky-smooth spreadable cheese that you can make sweet or savory for a meal or snack. One of my favorite ways to use it is simple: Spread it on high-fiber whole-grain toast and top it with fruit. Perfect for a quick breakfast or afternoon snack.

4 slices of whole-grain bread

½ cup ricotta cheese (whole milk or low fat)

1 tablespoon honey

Sea salt

1 cup fresh strawberries, sliced

4 large fresh basil leaves, sliced into thin shreds

1. Toast the bread.

2. In a small bowl, combine the ricotta, honey, and a pinch or two of sea salt. Taste and add additional honey or salt if desired.

3. Spread the mixture evenly over each slice of bread (about 2 tablespoons per slice).

4. Top each piece with sliced strawberries and a few pieces of shredded basil.

INGREDIENT TIP: When buying bread, always look for "whole grain" or "100% whole wheat" on the label. It has more fiber and nutrients.

VARIATION TIP: Try a savory version of this recipe by skipping the honey in the ricotta cheese and substituting sliced cucumbers for the strawberries.

Per Serving: Calories: 275; Total fat: 8g; Total carbs: 41g; Fiber: 5g; Sugar: 16g; Protein: 15g; Sodium: 323mg; Cholesterol: 19mg

CHERRY ALMOND BAKED OATMEAL CUPS

Prep Time: 10 minutes, plus 10 minutes to cool / Cook Time: 35–45 minutes / Serves 2
gluten-free, vegetarian

Oats are one of the best whole grains you can eat to help lower your cholesterol. They're packed with soluble fiber, which reduces your LDL ("bad") cholesterol. It also helps to stabilize your blood sugar and keep you feeling full for longer. Plus, baked oats make the house smell wonderful!

½ cup gluten-free old-fashioned oats

2 tablespoons sliced almonds

Pinch salt

¾ cup milk

½ teaspoon almond extract

½ teaspoon vanilla

1 egg, beaten

2 tablespoons maple syrup

1 cup frozen cherries, thawed

Ricotta cheese (optional, for topping)

Greek yogurt (optional, for topping)

1. Preheat the oven to 350°F and set the rack to the middle position. Oil two 8-ounce ramekins and place them on a baking sheet.

2. In a medium bowl, combine all of the ingredients and mix well.

3. Spoon half of the mixture into each ramekin.

4. Bake for 35 to 45 minutes, or until the oats are set and a knife inserted into the middle comes out clean. They will be soft but should not be runny.

5. Let the baked oats cool for 5 to 10 minutes. Top with ricotta cheese or plain Greek yogurt, if desired.

PREP TIP: If time is short in the morning, you can bake these up the night before and just reheat them in the microwave when you're ready for breakfast. You can also double this recipe easily and prepare it in a baking dish if you want enough for several days.

INGREDIENT TIP: Frozen berries work well here, too. I always keep bags of frozen fruit in my freezer for recipes like this.

Per Serving: Calories: 287; Total fat: 9g; Total carbs: 43g; Fiber: 4g; Sugar: 24g; Protein: 11g; Sodium: 155mg; Cholesterol: 89mg

INDIVIDUAL BAKED EGG CASSEROLES

Prep Time: 10 minutes / Cook Time: 30 minutes / Serves 2
vegetarian

In case you were wondering . . . eggs are back on the *Do Eat* list! The yolks don't raise your cholesterol (it's the butter and bacon that do that!) and in fact, they're a good source of protein, healthy fats, vitamin D, choline, and antioxidants. Eggs also pair nicely with vegetables, which makes them perfect for any meal.

1 slice whole-grain bread

4 large eggs, beaten

3 tablespoons milk

¼ teaspoon salt

½ teaspoon onion powder

¼ teaspoon garlic powder

Pinch freshly ground black pepper

¾ cup chopped vegetables (any kind you like—e.g., cherry tomatoes, mushrooms, scallions, spinach, broccoli, etc.)

1. Heat the oven to 375°F and set the rack to the middle position. Oil two 8-ounce ramekins and place them on a baking sheet.

2. Tear the bread into pieces and line each ramekin with ½ of a slice.

3. Mix the eggs, milk, salt, onion powder, garlic powder, pepper, and vegetables in a medium bowl.

4. Pour half of the egg mixture into each ramekin.

5. Bake for 30 minutes, or until the eggs are set.

PREP TIP: You can prep these the night before and bake them in the morning. If you have leftover vegetables from dinner, save them to use in this recipe.

VARIATION TIP: Feel free to add meat or cheese to the mixture.

Per Serving: Calories: 213; Total fat: 12g; Total carbs: 13g; Fiber: 2g; Sugar: 4g; Protein: 17g; Sodium: 518mg; Cholesterol: 374mg

OVERNIGHT POMEGRANATE MUESLI

Prep Time: 10 minutes, plus overnight to chill / Serves 2
30 minutes, gluten-free, vegetarian

Muesli is the European version of overnight oats. It's lower in sugar than American-style oats, and it's kicked up with lots of nuts, seeds, and some yogurt for extra healthy fats and protein. I eat some version of this quite often for breakfast, and I love that you can make it the night before. When the oats soak in the milk, they soften just as they would if they were cooked. If you can find the thick-cut oats, use them here—they provide a wonderful, hearty texture.

½ cup gluten-free old-fashioned oats

¼ cup shelled pistachios

3 tablespoons pumpkin seeds

2 tablespoons chia seeds

¾ cup milk

½ cup plain Greek yogurt

2 to 3 teaspoons maple syrup (optional)

½ cup pomegranate arils

1. In a medium bowl, mix together the oats, pistachios, pumpkin seeds, chia seeds, milk, yogurt, and maple syrup, if using.

2. Divide the mixture between two 12-ounce mason jars or another type of container with a lid.

3. Top each with ¼ cup of pomegranate arils.

4. Cover each jar or container and store in the refrigerator overnight or up to 4 days.

5. Serve cold, with additional milk if desired.

SUBSTITUTION TIP: If pomegranates aren't in season, you can substitute fresh or frozen berries.

VARIATION TIP: Make this nondairy by substituting plant-based milk and yogurt.

Per Serving: Calories: 502; Total fat: 24g; Total carbs: 60g; Fiber: 10g; Sugar: 33g; Protein: 17g; Sodium: 171mg; Cholesterol: 20mg

MEDITERRANEAN BREAKFAST PIZZA

Prep Time: 5 minutes / Cook Time: 15 minutes / Serves 2

30 minutes, vegetarian

This is not your average cold leftover pizza for breakfast! With this breakfast pizza you can start your day with some vegetables and protein so you'll stay full and satisfied until lunch. Tomatoes are rich in lycopene, an antioxidant that protects your heart and may reduce the risk of some types of cancer. When you combine tomatoes with some olive oil (as I do here with the pesto) your body absorbs more of that lycopene.

2 (6- to 8-inch-long) pieces of whole-wheat naan bread

2 tablespoons prepared pesto

1 medium tomato, sliced

2 large eggs

1. Heat a large nonstick skillet over medium-high heat. Place the naan bread in the skillet and let it warm for about 2 minutes on each side. The bread should be softened and just starting to turn golden.

2. Spread 1 tablespoon of the pesto on one side of each slice. Top the pesto with tomato slices to cover. Remove the pizzas from the pan and place each one on its own plate.

3. Crack the eggs into the pan, keeping them separated, and cook until the whites are no longer translucent and the yolk is cooked to desired doneness.

4. With a spatula, spoon one egg onto each pizza.

PREP TIP: If the fresh basil in your garden is growing out of control, make a big batch of pesto and freeze it in an ice cube tray. Those individual portions are perfect for a recipe like this.

INGREDIENT TIP: When buying prepared pesto, look for one that's made with heart-healthy olive oil or canola oil, and skip those with soybean oil.

Per Serving: Calories: 427; Total fat: 17g; Total carbs: 10g; Fiber: 5g; Sugar: 4g; Protein: 17g; Sodium: 718mg; Cholesterol: 188mg

TOMATO GOAT CHEESE STOVETOP FRITTATA

Prep Time: 15 minutes / Cook Time: 25 minutes / Serves 2

gluten-free, vegetarian

Frittatas are a great "back pocket" meal—they need minimal prep and come together quickly with whatever you have on hand. They're great for breakfast, or even a quick dinner, and leftovers are perfect for another meal. Traditionally, frittatas are finished in an oven, where they get puffed and golden, but when time is short, a stovetop works well too. Use a small pan for a thicker frittata, or a larger pan for more of an omelet-style frittata.

1 tablespoon olive oil

½ pint cherry or grape tomatoes

2 garlic cloves, minced

5 large eggs, beaten

3 tablespoons milk

½ teaspoon salt

Pinch freshly ground black pepper

2 tablespoons minced fresh oregano

2 tablespoons minced fresh basil

2 ounces crumbled goat cheese (about ½ cup)

1. Heat the oil in a nonstick skillet over medium heat. Add the tomatoes. As they start to cook, pierce some of them so they give off some of their juice. Reduce the heat to medium-low, cover the pan, and let the tomatoes soften.

2. When the tomatoes are mostly softened and broken down, remove the lid, add the garlic and continue to sauté.

3. In a medium bowl, combine the eggs, milk, salt, pepper, and herbs and whisk well to combine.

4. Turn the heat up to medium-high. Add the egg mixture to the tomatoes and garlic, then sprinkle the goat cheese over the eggs.

5. Cover the pan and let cook for about 7 minutes.

6. Uncover the pan and continue cooking for another 7 to 10 minutes, or until the eggs are set. Run a spatula around the edge of the pan to make sure they won't stick.

7. Let the frittata cool for about 5 minutes before serving. Cut it into wedges and serve.

PREP TIP: Make this the night before and eat it cold, at room temperature, or reheated for breakfast the next morning.

INGREDIENT TIP: If you don't have fresh herbs available, substitute dried herbs.

Per Serving: Calories: 417; Total fat: 31g; Total carbs: 12g; Fiber: 3g; Sugar: 6g; Protein: 26g; Sodium: 867mg; Cholesterol: 497mg

SHAKSHUKA

Prep Time: 15 minutes / Cook Time: 30 minutes / Serves 2
gluten-free, vegetarian

Shakshuka is a traditional North African (Tunisian) breakfast that also works for a quick and easy dinner. It's packed with disease-fighting antioxidants from the spices, tomatoes, and sweet peppers, and even the eggs have antioxidants in the yolks.

1 tablespoon olive oil

½ **red pepper, diced (about ½ cup)**

½ **medium onion, diced (about ½ cup)**

2 small garlic cloves, minced

½ teaspoon cumin

½ teaspoon smoked paprika

Pinch red pepper flakes (more or less to taste)

1 (14.5-ounce) can fire-roasted tomatoes

¼ teaspoon salt

Pinch freshly ground black pepper

1 ounce crumbled feta cheese (about ¼ cup)

3 large eggs

3 tablespoons minced fresh parsley

Pita chips or pita bread to serve

1. Heat the olive oil in a skillet over medium-high heat and add the pepper, onion, and garlic. Sauté until the vegetables start to turn golden.

2. Add the cumin, paprika, and red pepper flakes and stir to toast the spices for about 30 seconds. Add the tomatoes with their juices.

3. Reduce the heat and let the sauce simmer for 10 minutes, or until it starts to thicken a bit. Add the salt and pepper. Taste the sauce and adjust seasonings as necessary.

4. Sprinkle the feta cheese on top.

5. Make 3 wells in the sauce and crack an egg into each well.

6. Cover the pan and let the eggs cook for about 7 minutes. Remove the lid and continue cooking for 5 more minutes, or until the yolks are cooked to desired doneness.

7. Garnish with fresh parsley.

8. If desired, serve with pita chips or bread to scoop up the sauce.

Per Serving: Calories: 287; Total fat: 18g; Total carbs: 18g; Fiber: 5g; Sugar: 9g; Protein: 14g; Sodium: 422mg; Cholesterol: 292mg

POWER PEACH SMOOTHIE BOWL

Prep Time: 15 minutes / Serves 2

30 minutes, gluten-free, vegetarian

A smoothie bowl is a thick smoothie that you eat with a spoon. This one features frozen peaches, which are available year-round. I often add avocado to a smoothie to provide additional creaminess and thickness. Even though it's not traditional to the Mediterranean diet, it's packed with the same heart-healthy fats as olives and olive oil. Customize your smoothie bowl by adding any of the following toppings: chia seeds, sunflower seeds, shredded unsweetened coconut, cocoa nibs, or chopped nuts.

2 cups packed partially thawed frozen peaches

½ cup plain or vanilla Greek yogurt

½ ripe avocado

2 tablespoons flax meal

1 teaspoon vanilla extract

1 teaspoon orange extract

1 tablespoon honey (optional)

1. Combine all of the ingredients in a blender and blend until smooth.

2. Pour the mixture into two bowls, and, if desired, sprinkle with additional toppings.

PREP TIP: To quickly thaw your peaches, microwave them in a microwave-safe glass measuring cup until they are mostly thawed, but still a bit frozen in the middle. To store your leftover avocado and keep it from browning, drizzle the cut side with some olive oil, wrap it tightly with plastic wrap, and store it in the refrigerator.

VARIATION TIP: If you prefer a drinkable smoothie, skip the Greek yogurt and add 1 cup of milk or unsweetened kefir, a probiotic yogurt drink.

Per Serving: Calories: 213; Total fat: 13g; Total carbs: 23g; Fiber: 7g; Sugar: 15g; Protein: 6g; Sodium: 41mg; Cholesterol: 13mg

SPINACH, SUN-DRIED TOMATO, AND FETA EGG WRAPS

Prep Time: 10 minutes / **Cook Time:** 7 minutes / **Serves 2**

30 minutes, vegetarian

Egg wraps are an easy way to turn scrambled eggs into a full, balanced meal. These hit all of the food groups, and they're a tasty way to start your day with a serving of vegetables.

1 tablespoon olive oil

¼ cup minced onion

3 to 4 tablespoons minced sun-dried tomatoes in olive oil and herbs

3 large eggs, beaten

1½ cups packed baby spinach

1 ounce crumbled feta cheese

Salt

2 (8-inch) whole-wheat tortillas

1. In a large skillet, heat the olive oil over medium-high heat. Add the onion and tomatoes and sauté for about 3 minutes.

2. Turn the heat down to medium. Add the beaten eggs and stir to scramble them.

3. Add the spinach and stir to combine. Sprinkle the feta cheese over the eggs. Add salt to taste.

4. Warm the tortillas in the microwave for about 20 seconds each.

5. Fill each tortilla with half of the egg mixture. Fold in half or roll them up and serve.

SUBSTITUTION TIP: If you prefer a spicier version, swap in a few teaspoons of harissa sauce for the sun-dried tomatoes.

INGREDIENT TIP: I always keep a jar of sun-dried tomatoes in olive oil and herbs in my refrigerator. They give almost any dish a pop of flavor.

Per Serving: Calories: 435; Total fat: 28g; Total carbs: 31g; Fiber: 6g; Sugar: 6g; Protein: 17g; Sodium: 552mg; Cholesterol: 292mg

SAVORY PARMESAN OATMEAL

Prep Time: 10 minutes / Cook Time: 20 minutes / Serves 2
30 minutes, gluten-free

This quick and easy recipe is proof that oats are a versatile whole grain that work as a savory meal too. Old-fashioned oats cook up in minutes, and much like rice or polenta, they're especially delicious with a sprinkle of Parmesan cheese.

1 tablespoon olive oil

¼ cup minced onion

1 ounce (about 2 thin slices) prosciutto, minced

2 cups greens (arugula, baby spinach, chopped kale, or Swiss chard)

¾ cup gluten-free old-fashioned oats

1½ cups water, unsalted, or low-sodium chicken stock

2 tablespoons Parmesan cheese

Salt

Pinch freshly ground black pepper

1. Heat the olive oil in a saucepan over medium-high heat. Add the onion and prosciutto and sauté for 4 minutes, or until the prosciutto starts to crisp and the onion turns golden.

2. Add the greens and stir until they begin to wilt. Transfer this mixture to a bowl.

3. Add the oats to the pan and let them toast for about 2 minutes. Add the water or chicken stock and bring the oats to a boil. Reduce the heat to low, cover the pan, and let the oats cook for 10 minutes, or until the liquid is absorbed and the oats are tender.

4. Stir the Parmesan cheese into the oats, and add the onions, prosciutto, and greens back to the pan. Add additional water if needed, so the oats are creamy and not dry.

5. Stir well and add salt and freshly ground black pepper to taste.

PREP TIP: If you don't have no- or low-sodium stock or broth, stick to water and add your own salt as needed. The cheese and prosciutto are quite high in salt, so regular stock makes this dish too salty.

Per Serving: Calories: 258; Total fat: 12g; Total carbs: 29g; Fiber: 6g; Sugar: 1g; Protein: 11g; Sodium: 260mg; Cholesterol: 13mg

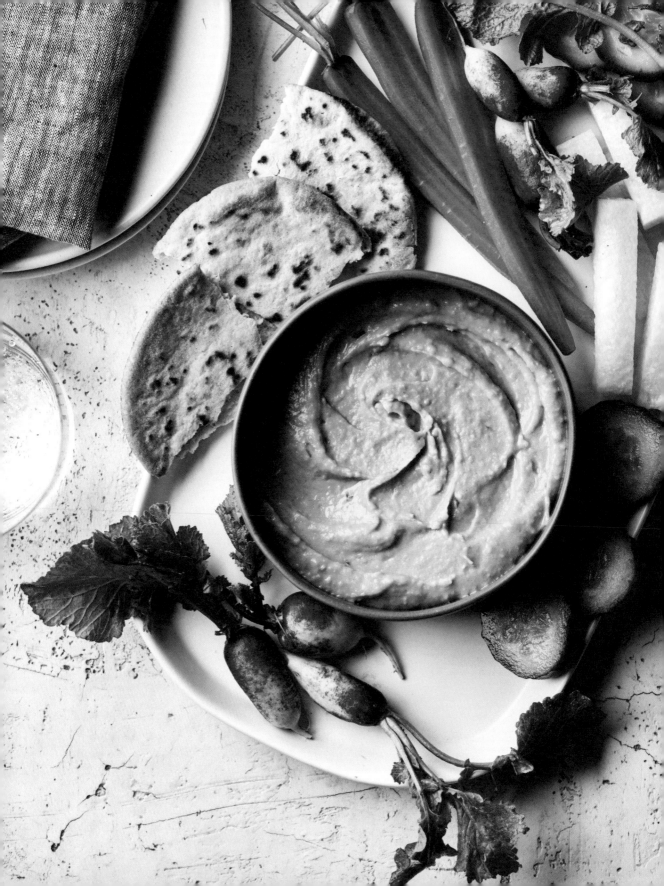

CHAPTER 4

SNACKS

Snacks are an important part of a healthy meal plan, and they should be every bit as balanced with protein, healthy fats, and high-fiber carbs as your meals. Eating smaller meals with a snack or two in between is a great strategy to maintain balanced blood sugar and a healthy weight, because it prevents you from overeating at the next meal.

To me, the true test of a good snack is whether it can stand alone as a mini meal. I can personally attest that each of the snacks I've included here can do that. And if you find yourself having one of those nights where you just don't feel like cooking dinner, just bump up the portion size on any of these—or combine a few snacks and call it a night!

< White Bean Harissa Dip, page 40

WHITE BEAN HARISSA DIP

Prep Time: 10 minutes / Cook Time: 1 hour / Makes 1½ cups

dairy-free, gluten-free, vegan, vegetarian

Beans are a staple in the Mediterranean diet. They're linked to reduced risk of heart disease, diabetes, and some forms of cancer. In addition to eating them whole, I like to have a container of white bean dip in the refrigerator for snacks with crackers, pita, or vegetables, or to spread on a sandwich. This one has a nice spicy kick from harissa, a Tunisian spice paste that you can find at specialty stores, Amazon, or Trader Joe's.

1 whole head of garlic

½ cup olive oil, divided

1 (15-ounce) can cannellini beans, drained and rinsed

1 teaspoon salt

1 teaspoon harissa paste (or more to taste)

1. Preheat the oven to 350°F.

2. Cut about ½ inch off the top of a whole head of garlic and lightly wrap it in foil. Drizzle 1 to 2 teaspoons of olive oil over the top of the cut side. Place it in an oven-safe dish and roast it in the oven for about 1 hour or until the cloves are soft and tender.

3. Remove the garlic from the oven and let it cool. The garlic can be roasted up to 2 days ahead of time.

4. Remove the garlic cloves from their skin and place them in the bowl of a food processor along with the beans, salt, and harissa. Purée, drizzling in as much olive oil as needed until the beans are smooth. If the dip seems too stiff, add additional olive oil to loosen the dip.

5. Taste the dip and add additional salt, harissa, or oil as needed.

6. Store in the refrigerator for up to a week.

7. Portion out ¼ cup of dip and serve with a mixture of raw vegetables and mini pita breads.

PREP TIP: Rather than heating up your oven for one head of garlic, keep an extra head or two of garlic on hand and roast it when you have your oven on for another meal. You can use roasted garlic the same way you use fresh or dried garlic, but it's so much sweeter and mellower.

VARIATION TIP: The beans, garlic, and olive oil are a blank slate for many flavors. Instead of the spicy harissa paste, try seasoning your dip with fresh rosemary, cumin, or a few sun-dried tomatoes.

Per Serving (¼ cup): Calories: 209; Total fat: 17g; Total carbs: 12g; Fiber: 3g; Sugar: 0g; Protein: 4g; Sodium: 389mg; Cholesterol: 0mg

MEDITERRANEAN TRAIL MIX

Prep Time: 10 minutes / Cook Time: 10 minutes / Makes 4 cups
30 minutes, dairy-free, gluten-free, vegan, vegetarian

Trail mix is the ultimate grab-and-go energy snack, whether you're hiking or running errands all day with no time for a meal. Nuts provide healthy fats, and they're an essential part of the Mediterranean diet. All types of nuts have health benefits, and eating them daily is linked with lower risk of heart disease, diabetes, and other chronic diseases. The key to eating nuts and trail mix is to limit the portion size to a handful, because they are high in calories.

1 tablespoon olive oil

1 tablespoon maple syrup

1 teaspoon vanilla

½ teaspoon cardamom

½ teaspoon allspice

2 cups mixed, unsalted nuts

¼ cup unsalted pumpkin or sunflower seeds

½ cup dried apricots, diced or thin sliced

½ cup dried figs, diced or thinly sliced

Pinch salt

1. Combine the olive oil, maple syrup, vanilla, cardamom, and allspice in a large sauté pan over medium heat. Stir to combine.

2. Add the nuts and seeds and stir well to coat. Let the nuts and seeds toast for about 10 minutes, stirring frequently.

3. Remove from the heat, and add the dried apricots and figs. Stir everything well and season with salt.

4. Store in an airtight container.

INGREDIENT TIP: Nuts are a great thing to buy in bulk. As long as you store them in airtight containers, they'll last for a few months. Look for raw nuts that don't have added salt or sugar. That way you can toast them and flavor them in any way you like.

Per Serving (½ cup): Calories: 261; Total fat: 18g; Total carbs: 23 g; Fiber: 5g; Sugar: 12g; Protein: 6g; Sodium: 26mg; Cholesterol: 0mg

SEARED HALLOUMI WITH PESTO AND TOMATO

Prep Time: 2 minutes / Cook Time: 5 minutes / Serves 2

30 minutes, gluten-free, vegetarian

The first time I had Halloumi was in a restaurant in Boston. I thought I was ordering fish—but Halloumi is a type of Greek cheese! It's deliciously salty and squeaks when you chew it. Halloumi is usually served seared or grilled. It gets warm and soft on the outside, but it doesn't fully melt.

3 ounces Halloumi cheese, cut crosswise into 2 thinner, rectangular pieces

2 teaspoons prepared pesto sauce, plus additional for drizzling if desired

1 medium tomato, sliced

1. Heat a nonstick skillet over medium-high heat and place the slices of Halloumi in the hot pan. After about 2 minutes, check to see if the cheese is golden on the bottom. If it is, flip the slices, top each with 1 teaspoon of pesto, and cook for another 2 minutes, or until the second side is golden.

2. Serve with slices of tomato and a drizzle of pesto, if desired, on the side.

PREP TIP: Because Halloumi is a fairly salty cheese, no additional salt is needed in this dish.

Per Serving: Calories: 177; Total fat: 14g; Total carbs: 4g; Fiber: 1g; Sugar: 3g; Protein: 10g; Sodium: 233mg; Cholesterol: 34mg

STUFFED CUCUMBER CUPS

Prep Time: 5 minutes / Serves 2

30 minutes, dairy-free, gluten-free, vegan, vegetarian

This couldn't be an easier recipe, and it's packed with fresh Mediterranean flavors. I love this as a snack, but cucumber cups are also a quick and healthy bite-size appetizer idea. Make these with any flavor of store-bought hummus and cherry tomatoes—or try it with the White Bean Harissa Dip (page 40), and a tiny spoonful of Greek salsa (Chicken Cutlets with Greek Salsa, page 112).

1 medium cucumber (about 8 ounces, 8 to 9 inches long)

½ cup hummus (any flavor) or white bean dip

4 or 5 cherry tomatoes, sliced in half

2 tablespoons fresh basil, minced

1. Slice the ends off the cucumber (about ½ inch from each side) and slice the cucumber into 1-inch pieces.

2. With a paring knife or a spoon, scoop most of the seeds from the inside of each cucumber piece to make a cup, being careful to not cut all the way through.

3. Fill each cucumber cup with about 1 tablespoon of hummus or bean dip.

4. Top each with a cherry tomato half and a sprinkle of fresh minced basil.

VARIATION TIP: Experiment with different toppings such as chopped olives, sun-dried tomatoes, or feta cheese instead of the cherry tomatoes and basil.

Per Serving: Calories: 135; Total fat: 6g; Total carbs: 16g; Fiber: 5g; Sugar: 4g; Protein: 6g; Sodium: 242mg; Cholesterol: 0mg

ARABIC-STYLE SPICED ROASTED CHICKPEAS

Prep Time: 15 minutes / Cook Time: 35 minutes / Serves 2

dairy-free, gluten-free, vegan, vegetarian

Chickpeas are packed with fiber and these have so many antioxidants from the Arabic-inspired spice mix—which is a perfect combination of spicy, savory, and sweet.

For the seasoning mix

¾ teaspoon cumin

½ teaspoon coriander

½ teaspoon salt

¼ teaspoon freshly ground black pepper

¼ teaspoon paprika

¼ teaspoon cardamom

¼ teaspoon cinnamon

¼ teaspoon allspice

For the chickpeas

1 (15-ounce) can chickpeas, drained and rinsed

1 tablespoon olive oil

¼ teaspoon salt

To make the seasoning mix

In a small bowl, combine the cumin, coriander, salt, freshly ground black pepper, paprika, cardamom, cinnamon, and allspice. Stir well to combine and set aside.

To make the chickpeas

1. Preheat the oven to 400°F and set the rack to the middle position. Line a baking sheet with parchment paper.

2. Pat the rinsed chickpeas with paper towels or roll them in a clean kitchen towel to dry off any water.

3. Place the chickpeas in a bowl and season them with the olive oil and salt.

4. Add the chickpeas to the lined baking sheet (reserve the bowl) and roast them for about 25 to 35 minutes, turning them over once or twice while cooking. Most should be light brown. Taste one or two to make sure they are slightly crisp.

5. Place the roasted chickpeas back into the bowl and sprinkle them with the seasoning mix. Toss lightly to combine. Taste, and add additional salt if needed. Serve warm.

Per Serving: Calories: 268; Total fat: 11g; Total carbs: 35g; Fiber: 10g; Sugar: 6g; Protein: 11g; Sodium: 301mg; Cholesterol: 0mg

APPLE CHIPS WITH CHOCOLATE TAHINI

Prep Time: 10 minutes / Serves 2

30 minutes, dairy-free, gluten-free, vegan, vegetarian

Tahini is the Mediterranean version of peanut butter: a creamy spread that's made from ground sesame seeds. It's extremely rich in heart-healthy unsaturated fats, and it's a nice change from peanut butter. The oil tends to separate from the paste, so make sure you stir it well before using.

2 tablespoons tahini

1 tablespoon maple syrup

1 tablespoon unsweetened cocoa powder

1 to 2 tablespoons warm water (or more if needed)

2 medium apples

1 tablespoon roasted, salted sunflower seeds

1. In a small bowl, mix together the tahini, maple syrup, and cocoa powder. Add warm water, a little at a time, until thin enough to drizzle. Do not microwave it to thin it—it won't work.

2. Slice the apples crosswise into round slices, and then cut each piece in half to make a chip.

3. Lay the apple chips out on a plate and drizzle them with the chocolate tahini sauce.

4. Sprinkle sunflower seeds over the apple chips.

SUBSTITUTION TIP: Any type of nut or seed butter works well here, so try it with peanut, almond, or even sunflower butter.

Per Serving: Calories: 261; Total fat: 11g; Total carbs: 43g; Fiber: 8g; Sugar: 29g; Protein: 5g; Sodium: 21mg; Cholesterol: 0mg

STRAWBERRY CAPRESE SKEWERS

Prep Time: 15 minutes / Serves 2

30 minutes, gluten-free, vegetarian

These skewers are a sweet version of the traditional tomato caprese salad. They're great for an easy everyday snack or a quick and colorful appetizer idea. You'll be surprised at how well strawberries pair with these savory flavors.

½ cup balsamic vinegar

16 whole, hulled strawberries

12 small basil leaves or 6 large leaves, halved

12 pieces of small mozzarella balls (ciliegine)

1. To make the balsamic glaze, pour the balsamic vinegar into a small saucepan and bring it to a boil. Reduce the heat to medium-low and simmer for 10 minutes, or until it's reduced by half and is thick enough to coat the back of a spoon.

2. On each of 4 wooden skewers, place a strawberry, a folded basil leaf, and a mozzarella ball, repeating twice and adding a strawberry on the end. (Each skewer should have 4 strawberries, 3 basil leaves, and 3 mozzarella balls.)

3. Drizzle 1 to 2 teaspoons of balsamic glaze over the skewers.

INGREDIENT TIPS: *Ciliegine* are tiny mozzarella balls, about the size of cherries ("ciliegine" means "cherries" in Italian). They're usually available in the gourmet cheese department of the grocery store. Bottled balsamic glaze is also readily available at most grocery stores, but look for one without added sugar. It's a great condiment to drizzle on salads, vegetables, or even fresh berries.

VARIATION TIP: Turn this into a salad by skipping the skewers and serving the sliced strawberries and mozzarella balls on a bed of baby spinach. Use the balsamic glaze and a drizzle of olive oil as a dressing.

Per Serving: Calories: 206; Total fat: 10g; Total carbs: 17g; Fiber: 1g; Sugar: 14g; Protein: 10g; Sodium: 282mg; Cholesterol: 34mg

HERBED LABNEH VEGETABLE PARFAITS

Prep Time: 15 minutes (plus overnight if making your own labneh) / Serves 2
gluten-free, vegetarian

Labneh is yogurt cheese, and one of my favorite versatile sweet or savory dip bases. It's similar to cream cheese, luscious, smooth, but a bit tangier since it's made from yogurt. Because it's full of probiotics, it's also healthier for you. You can buy labneh at some natural food stores, but it's very easy to make your own. Za'atar is a classic Middle Eastern spice mix that pairs well with labneh for a savory snack.

For the labneh

8 ounces plain Greek yogurt (full fat works best)

Generous pinch salt

1 teaspoon za'atar seasoning

1 teaspoon freshly squeezed lemon juice

Pinch lemon zest

For the parfaits

½ cup peeled, chopped cucumber

½ cup grated carrots

½ cup cherry tomatoes, halved

To make the labneh

1. Line a strainer with cheesecloth and place it over a bowl.

2. Stir together the Greek yogurt and salt and place in the cheesecloth. Wrap it up and let it sit for 24 hours in the refrigerator.

3. When ready, unwrap the labneh and place it into a clean bowl. Stir in the za'atar, lemon juice, and lemon zest.

To make the parfaits

1. Divide the cucumber between two clear glasses.

2. Top each portion of cucumber with about 3 tablespoons of labneh.

3. Divide the carrots between the glasses.

4. Top with another 3 tablespoons of the labneh.

5. Top parfaits with the cherry tomatoes.

INGREDIENT TIP: Za'atar is a spice blend that often includes oregano, thyme, marjoram, sesame seeds, and sumac. It's available in the spice section of many grocery stores, or you can order it from a spice shop like Penzeys or Spicely.

PREP TIP: Double or triple the basic labneh recipe if you like. It keeps for about a week in the refrigerator.

Per Serving: Calories: 143; Total fat: 7g; Total carbs: 16g; Fiber: 2g; Sugar: 13g; Protein: 5g; Sodium: 187mg; Cholesterol: 25mg

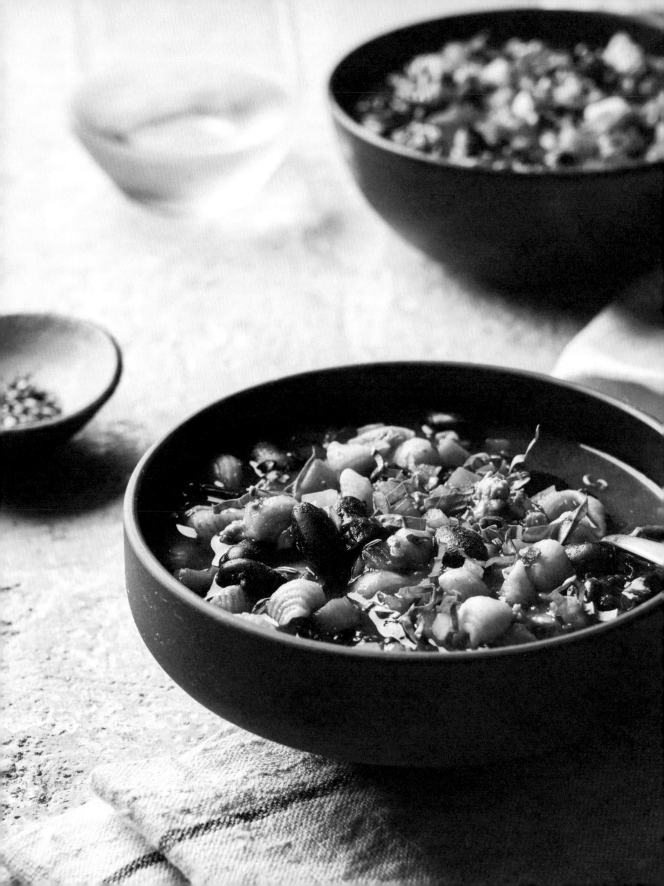

CHAPTER 5

SOUPS AND SALADS

It never ceases to amaze me how many flavorful combinations exist for soup and salad. I especially enjoy making them because it's a great chance to experiment with different seasonings and ingredients—and they're so forgiving. A little more of this or less of that, depending on your taste preferences, and you'll still have a great meal in the end.

And, let's not forget that both soups and salads are jam-packed with the healthiest foods on the planet in each and every bite. Both are a delicious way to enjoy the goodness of the Mediterranean diet.

Because I think soup always tastes better the next day, these soup recipes make four servings instead of two. You can eat the leftovers for lunch or dinner the next day, or freeze them for a later date.

< Hearty Italian Turkey Vegetable Soup, page 52

HEARTY ITALIAN TURKEY VEGETABLE SOUP

Prep Time: 30 minutes / Cook Time: 1 hour 10 minutes / Serves 2, with 2 servings for leftovers

dairy-free

Fennel is native to the Mediterranean region, and it adds such a wonderful, fresh, spicy-sweet flavor to this soup. I love it so much I use both the bulb and fennel seeds here. Fennel is especially helpful for digestion, and it's packed with potassium, which helps lower blood pressure.

1 tablespoon olive oil

½ pound lean ground turkey

1 celery stalk, diced (about ¼ cup)

2 medium carrots, diced (about ¾ cup)

1 small onion, diced (about 1 cup)

1 small fennel bulb, diced (about 1 cup)

1 garlic clove, minced

1 large leaf lacinato (dinosaur) kale, stemmed and chopped

2½ cups low-sodium tomato juice (not V8 juice)

2 cups low-sodium chicken stock

1 (15-ounce) can kidney beans, drained and rinsed

¾ teaspoon fennel seeds

¼ teaspoon red pepper flakes (optional)

¾ cup small shell pasta

2 tablespoons fresh basil, thinly sliced (about 4 basil leaves)

Salt

1. Heat the olive oil in a stockpot over medium-high heat. Add the turkey and sauté for 10 minutes, or until it's no longer pink.

2. Add the celery, carrots, onion, fennel, garlic, and kale and sauté for about 10 minutes.

3. Add the tomato juice, chicken stock, kidney beans, fennel seeds, and red pepper flakes and bring the soup to a boil. Reduce the heat, cover the pot, and let the soup simmer for 40 minutes, or until the carrots are softened.

4. Add the pasta and cook for another 10 minutes, or until al dente.

5. Add the basil, and season with salt to taste—start with about ½ teaspoon.

Per Serving: Calories: 345; Total fat: 9g; Total carbs: 47g; Fiber: 11g; Sugar: 8g; Protein: 24g; Sodium: 588mg; Cholesterol: 53mg

CREAMY TOMATO HUMMUS SOUP

Prep Time: 10 minutes / Cook Time: 10 minutes / Serves 2, with 2 servings for leftovers

30 minutes, dairy-free, gluten-free

If you shy away from making soups because you feel they take too much time, this one's for you! Just three main ingredients, and dinner is done in a snap. My secret nondairy ingredient for making a flavorful, rich, and creamy soup is hummus. It's already full of flavor, so it saves you the steps of mincing garlic and measuring spices.

1 (14.5-ounce) can crushed tomatoes with basil

1 cup roasted red pepper hummus

2 cups low-sodium chicken stock

Salt

¼ cup fresh basil leaves, thinly sliced (optional, for garnish)

Garlic croutons (optional, for garnish)

1. Combine the canned tomatoes, hummus, and chicken stock in a blender and blend until smooth. Pour the mixture into a saucepan and bring it to a boil.

2. Season with salt and fresh basil if desired. Serve with garlic croutons as a garnish, if desired.

VARIATION TIP: To make this a heartier soup, add shredded chicken and precooked brown rice or barley.

Per Serving: Calories: 148; Total fat: 6g; Total carbs: 19g; Fiber: 4g; Sugar: 7g; Protein: 5g; Sodium: 680mg; Cholesterol: 0mg

SPICY SAUSAGE LENTIL SOUP

Prep Time: 30 minutes / Cook Time: 60 minutes / Serves 2, with 2 servings for leftovers
dairy-free, gluten-free

Soups have tremendous healing properties, and not just when you feel a cold coming on. Research suggests capsaicin, the compound in spicy red pepper, may help to boost your metabolism a bit. The lycopene, lutein, and beta-carotene in red, orange, and green vegetables are great for your skin, brain, and eyes. And, the soluble fiber in lentils helps stabilize your blood sugar. This soup has it all—and the spiciness definitely helps with congestion.

1 tablespoon olive oil

½ medium onion, diced (about ¾ cup)

2 links (8 ounces) spicy Italian sausage (turkey or pork), removed from casing

2 medium carrots, sliced into coins (about ¾ cup)

1 medium celery stalk, diced (about ¼ cup)

2 garlic cloves, minced

¼ teaspoon red pepper flakes (omit or use less if you prefer less spicy)

½ teaspoon thyme

1 teaspoon oregano

1 bay leaf

3 cups low-sodium chicken stock

1 (28-ounce) can crushed tomatoes

¾ cup brown lentils

1 cup packed baby spinach, sliced

½ teaspoon salt, plus more to taste

1. Heat the oil in a stockpot over medium-high heat. Add the onion and sausage and sauté, breaking up the sausage into small pieces.

2. Add the carrots, celery, and garlic, and continue to sauté for about 10 more minutes.

3. Add the red pepper flakes, thyme, oregano, bay leaf, chicken stock, and tomatoes. Bring the soup to a boil.

4. Reduce the heat to medium-low and add the lentils. Stir everything well, cover, and let the soup simmer for 45 minutes, or until the lentils and carrots are tender.

5. Remove the bay leaf. Add the spinach and season with salt—start with ½ teaspoon and add additional salt to taste.

SUBSTITUTION TIP: If you have any other greens, like kale or Swiss chard on hand, you can toss them in as well, or substitute them for the spinach.

Per Serving: Calories: 354; Total fat: 9g; Total carbs: 45g; Fiber: 12g; Sugar: 13g; Protein: 25g; Sodium: 694mg; Cholesterol: 17mg

VEGETABLE FAGIOLI

Prep Time: 30 minutes / Cook Time: 60 minutes / Serves 2, with 2 servings for leftovers

dairy-free, gluten-free, vegan, vegetarian

"Fagioli" is Italian for beans, and they're definitely the star of this soup. Beans are an essential part of the Mediterranean diet. They're also inexpensive, versatile to cook with, and highly nutritious. Even though they're high in carbs, beans have a low glycemic index, which means that they help to stabilize your blood sugar. The fiber in beans is also a natural cholesterol-buster.

1 tablespoon olive oil

2 medium carrots, diced (about ¾ cup)

2 medium celery stalks, diced (about ½ cup)

½ medium onion, diced (about ¾ cup)

1 large garlic clove, minced

3 tablespoons tomato paste

4 cups low-sodium vegetable broth

1 cup packed kale, stemmed and chopped

1 (15-ounce) can red kidney beans, drained and rinsed

1 (15-ounce) can cannellini beans, drained and rinsed

½ cup fresh basil, chopped

Salt

Freshly ground black pepper

1. Heat the olive oil in a stockpot over medium-high heat. Add the carrots, celery, onion, and garlic and sauté for 10 minutes, or until the vegetables start to turn golden.

2. Stir in the tomato paste and cook for about 30 seconds.

3. Add the vegetable broth and bring the soup to a boil. Cover, and reduce the heat to low. Cook the soup for 45 minutes, or until the carrots are tender.

4. Using an immersion blender, purée the soup so that it's partly smooth, but with some chunks of vegetables. If you don't have an immersion blender, scoop out about ⅓ of the soup and blend it in a blender, then add it back to the pot.

5. Add the kale, beans, and basil. Season with salt and pepper.

INGREDIENT TIP: For recipes that call for a small amount of tomato paste, buy the kind that comes in a tube instead of a can. You can squeeze out just the amount needed, and the tube can be stored in the refrigerator for a fairly long time.

Per Serving: Calories: 215; Total fat: 4g; Total carbs: 36g; Fiber: 11g; Sugar: 5g; Protein: 11g; Sodium: 486mg; Cholesterol: 0mg

AVGOLEMONO (LEMON CHICKEN SOUP)

Prep Time: 15 minutes / Cook Time: 60 minutes / Serves 2, with 2 servings for leftovers
dairy-free, gluten-free

Nearly every culture has their own version of chicken soup, and avgolemono is Greece's take on this classic. It features a bright pop of flavor from fresh lemon juice, combined with an egg yolk to thicken and enrich the soup. Avgolemono is a perfect soup to take away the chill if you feel a cold coming on. The lemon juice also provides vitamin C to boost your immune system.

½ large onion

2 medium carrots

1 celery stalk

1 garlic clove

5 cups low-sodium chicken stock

¼ cup brown rice

1½ cups (about 5 ounces) shredded rotisserie chicken

3 tablespoons freshly squeezed lemon juice

1 egg yolk

2 tablespoons chopped fresh dill

2 tablespoons chopped fresh parsley

Salt

1. Place the onion, carrots, celery, and garlic in a food processor fitted with the chopping blade and pulse it until the vegetables are minced. You can also mince them by hand.

2. Add the vegetables and chicken stock to a stockpot or Dutch oven and bring it to a boil over high heat.

3. Reduce the heat to medium-low and add the rice, shredded chicken and lemon juice. Cover, and let the soup simmer for 40 minutes, or until the rice is cooked.

4. In a small bowl, whisk the egg yolk lightly. Very slowly, while whisking with one hand, pour about ½ of a ladle of the broth into the egg yolk to warm, or temper, the yolk. Slowly add another ladle of broth and continue to whisk. Do not skip this step (see Prep Tip).

5. Remove the soup from the heat and pour the whisked egg yolk–broth mixture into the pot. Stir well to combine.

6. Add the fresh dill and parsley. Season with salt, and serve.

7. If you want to reheat any leftovers, heat it very slowly and don't let the soup come to a full boil.

PREP TIP: The proteins in ingredients like eggs (or yogurt) can cook or curdle if they're added directly to hot soup stock. By gently adding a small amount of hot liquid and whisking it in, you'll warm the egg yolks so they'll be more stable when they get mixed into the soup.

Per Serving: Calories: 171; Total fat: 3g; Total carbs: 16g; Fiber: 2g; Sugar: 3g; Protein: 19g; Sodium: 236mg; Cholesterol: 93mg

SIMPLE INSALATA MISTA (MIXED SALAD) WITH HONEY BALSAMIC DRESSING

Prep Time: 15 minutes / Serves 2

30 minutes, dairy-free, gluten-free, vegetarian

There's something magical about chopping up your salad ingredients and tossing them with dressing that just makes it taste better than a salad with large pieces of vegetables and dressing sitting on top. If you haven't tried this simple trick, I promise it's a game changer that will have you loving salad so much more.

For the dressing

¼ cup balsamic vinegar

¼ cup olive oil

1 tablespoon honey

1 teaspoon Dijon mustard

¼ teaspoon salt, plus more to taste

¼ teaspoon garlic powder

Pinch freshly ground black pepper

For the salad

4 cups chopped red leaf lettuce

½ cup cherry or grape tomatoes, halved

½ English cucumber, sliced in quarters lengthwise and then cut into bite-size pieces

Any combination fresh, torn herbs (parsley, oregano, basil, chives, etc.)

1 tablespoon roasted sunflower seeds

To make the dressing

Combine the vinegar, olive oil, honey, mustard, salt, garlic powder, and pepper in a jar with a lid. Shake well.

To make the salad

1. In a large bowl, combine the lettuce, tomatoes, cucumber, and herbs.

2. Toss well to combine.

3. Pour all or as much dressing as desired over the tossed salad and toss again to coat the salad with dressing.

4. Top with the sunflower seeds.

PREP TIP: I like to double or triple this dressing recipe, so I always have a jar in the refrigerator. It's so easy to make and tastes better than most bottled brands. And have you ever noticed that most bottled salad dressings contain little or no olive oil? They all use a less expensive (and less healthy) oil.

Per Serving: Calories: 339; Total fat: 26g; Total carbs: 24g; Fiber: 3g; Sugar: 17g; Protein: 4g; Sodium: 171mg; Cholesterol: 0mg

FIG AND ARUGULA SALAD

Prep Time: 15 minutes / Serves 2

30 minutes, gluten-free

Sweet figs and peppery arugula are two treasures from the Mediterranean region that were meant to be together—especially when paired with the other ingredients in this simple but satisfying salad, which is perfect for a side dish or a light meal. Arugula is a member of the cruciferous family of vegetables, full of antioxidants and compounds that have strong anticancer properties. Figs are rich in fiber, vitamins, and minerals, including potassium, which reduces blood pressure.

3 cups arugula

4 fresh, ripe figs (or 4 to 6 dried figs), stemmed and sliced

2 tablespoons olive oil

3 very thin slices prosciutto, trimmed of any fat and sliced lengthwise into 1-inch strips

¼ cup pecan halves, lightly toasted

2 tablespoons crumbled blue cheese

1 to 2 tablespoons balsamic glaze (see Strawberry Caprese Skewers, page 47)

1. In a large bowl, toss the arugula and figs with the olive oil.

2. Place the prosciutto on a microwave-safe plate and heat it on high in the microwave for 60 seconds, or until it just starts to crisp.

3. Add the crisped prosciutto, pecans, and blue cheese to the bowl. Toss the salad lightly.

4. Drizzle with the balsamic glaze.

INGREDIENT TIP: Fresh figs are in season from June through September, but dried, unsweetened figs are available year-round.

Per Serving: Calories: 519; Total fat: 38g; Total carbs: 30g; Fiber: 6g; Sugar: 24g; Protein: 20g; Sodium: 482mg; Cholesterol: 51mg

SUMMER PANZANELLA SALAD

Prep Time: 15 minutes / Cook Time: 10 minutes, plus 15 minutes to rest / Serves 2
vegetarian

One of the things I love best about the Mediterranean diet is the simplicity of its ingredients and how much the flavors of very fresh, seasonal foods shine. This salad is a perfect example. It's bursting with fresh flavor and gorgeous colors. Make it when it's corn season. If it's not in season, it's better to skip the corn than use frozen or canned corn.

Cooking spray

1 ear corn on the cob, peeled and shucked

4 slices stale French baguette

½ pint cherry or grape tomatoes, halved

1 medium sweet pepper, seeded and cut into 1-inch pieces

1 medium avocado, pitted and cut into cubes

4 very thin slices of sweet onion, cut crosswise into thin rings

½ cup fresh whole basil leaves

2 ounces mini mozzarella balls (ciliegine), halved or quartered

¼ cup honey balsamic dressing (see Simple Insalata Mista, page 58)

1. Heat the grill to medium-high heat (about 350°F) and lightly spray the cooking grates with cooking spray.

2. Grill the corn for 10 minutes, or until it is lightly charred all around.

3. Grill the bread for 30 to 45 seconds on each side, or until it has grill marks.

4. Let the corn sit until it's cool enough to handle. Cut the kernels off the cob and place them in a large bowl.

5. Cut the bread into chunks and add it to the bowl.

6. Add the tomatoes, sweet pepper, avocado, onion, basil, mozzarella, and dressing to the bowl, and toss lightly to combine. Let the salad sit for about 15 minutes in the refrigerator, so the bread can soften and the flavors can blend.

7. This is best served shortly after it's prepared.

INGREDIENT TIP: Any color sweet pepper works fine in this recipe, but I like to use orange, so I have as many different colors as possible. We eat with our eyes, after all!

Per Serving: Calories: 525; Total fat: 26g; Total carbs: 61g; Fiber: 10g; Sugar: 17g; Protein: 16g; Sodium: 524mg; Cholesterol: 19mg

WATERMELON FETA SALAD

Prep Time: 10 minutes / Serves 2

30 minutes, gluten-free, vegetarian

Watermelon's beautiful salmon-red color is a telltale sign that it's packed with antioxidants. It's especially rich in a carotene called lycopene, the compound that's linked with lower prostate cancer risk and reduced risk of heart disease, diabetes, and neurodegenerative diseases. Lycopene may also provide your skin protection from sunlight and UV rays. The first time I was introduced to the combination of watermelon and feta cheese, I'll admit I was skeptical, but trust me—it works.

3 cups packed arugula

2½ cups watermelon, cut into bite-size cubes

2 ounces feta cheese, crumbled

2 tablespoons balsamic glaze (see Strawberry Caprese Skewers, page 47)

1. Divide the arugula between two plates.

2. Divide the watermelon cubes between the beds of arugula.

3. Sprinkle 1 ounce of the feta over each salad.

4. Drizzle about 1 tablespoon of the glaze (or more if desired) over each salad.

PREP TIP: I don't think this salad needs any salt because the feta is salty enough, but feel free to add a pinch if you like.

Per Serving: Calories: 159; Total fat: 7g; Total carbs: 21g; Fiber: 1g; Sugar: 17g; Protein: 6g; Sodium: 327mg; Cholesterol: 25mg

GREEN BEAN AND HALLOUMI SALAD

Prep Time: 20 minutes / Cook Time: 5 minutes / Serves 2

30 minutes, gluten-free, vegetarian

I love to use kefir to make a creamy dressing. It's a tangy, slightly thick fermented milk that's full of probiotics. You can usually find it near the yogurt at the grocery store, but if you can't, buttermilk is a good substitute.

For the dressing

¼ cup plain kefir
or buttermilk

1 tablespoon olive oil

2 teaspoons freshly
squeezed lemon juice

¼ teaspoon
onion powder

¼ teaspoon garlic powder

Pinch salt

Pinch freshly ground
black pepper

For the salad

½ pound very fresh green
beans, trimmed

2 ounces Halloumi
cheese, sliced into
2 (½-inch-thick) slices

½ cup cherry or grape
tomatoes, halved

¼ cup very thinly sliced
sweet onion

2 ounces prosciutto,
cooked crisp
and crumbled

To make the dressing
Combine the kefir or buttermilk, olive oil, lemon juice, onion powder, garlic powder, salt, and pepper in a small bowl and whisk well. Set the dressing aside.

To make the salad
1. Fill a medium-size pot with about 1 inch of water and add the green beans. Cover and steam them for about 3 to 4 minutes, or just until beans are tender. Do not overcook. Drain beans, rinse them immediately with cold water, and set them aside to cool.

2. Heat a nonstick skillet over medium-high heat and place the slices of Halloumi in the hot pan. After about 2 minutes, check to see if the cheese is golden on the bottom. If it is, flip the slices and cook for another minute or until the second side is golden.

3. Remove cheese from the pan and cut each piece into cubes (about 1-inch square)

4. Place the green beans, halloumi, tomatoes, and sliced onion in a large bowl and toss to combine.

5. Drizzle dressing over the salad and toss well to combine. Sprinkle prosciutto over the top.

Per Serving: Calories: 273; Total fat: 18g; Total carbs: 16g; Fiber: 5g; Sugar: 7g; Protein: 15g; Sodium: 506mg; Cholesterol: 39mg

CITRUS FENNEL SALAD

Prep Time: 15 minutes / Serves 2

30 minutes, gluten-free, vegetarian

This salad is gorgeous when blood oranges are in season, but regular navel oranges work well too. Not only is it full of fresh flavors and aromas, it's also packed with potassium-rich ingredients excellent for managing blood pressure.

For the dressing

2 tablespoons fresh orange juice

3 tablespoons olive oil

1 tablespoon blood orange vinegar, other orange vinegar, or cider vinegar

1 tablespoon honey

Salt

Freshly ground black pepper

For the salad

2 cups packed baby kale

1 medium navel or blood orange, segmented

½ small fennel bulb, stems and leaves removed, sliced into matchsticks

3 tablespoons toasted pecans, chopped

2 ounces goat cheese, crumbled

To make the dressing

Combine the orange juice, olive oil, vinegar, and honey in a small bowl and whisk to combine. Season with salt and pepper. Set the dressing aside.

To make the salad

1. Divide the baby kale, orange segments, fennel, pecans, and goat cheese evenly between two plates.

2. Drizzle half of the dressing over each salad.

INGREDIENT TIP: Baby kale is usually sold prewashed in bags. If it's only available mixed with other greens, that works fine.

SUBSTITUTION TIP: If you want to substitute curly or lacinato (dinosaur) kale instead of baby kale, remove any tough stems, sprinkle it with salt and olive oil, and give it a good massage. Kale leaves are tough and sometimes bitter when eaten raw, but massaging them with oil and salt helps to soften them.

Per Serving: Calories: 502; Total fat: 39g; Total carbs: 31g; Fiber: 6g; Sugar: 17g; Protein: 13g; Sodium: 158mg; Cholesterol: 30mg

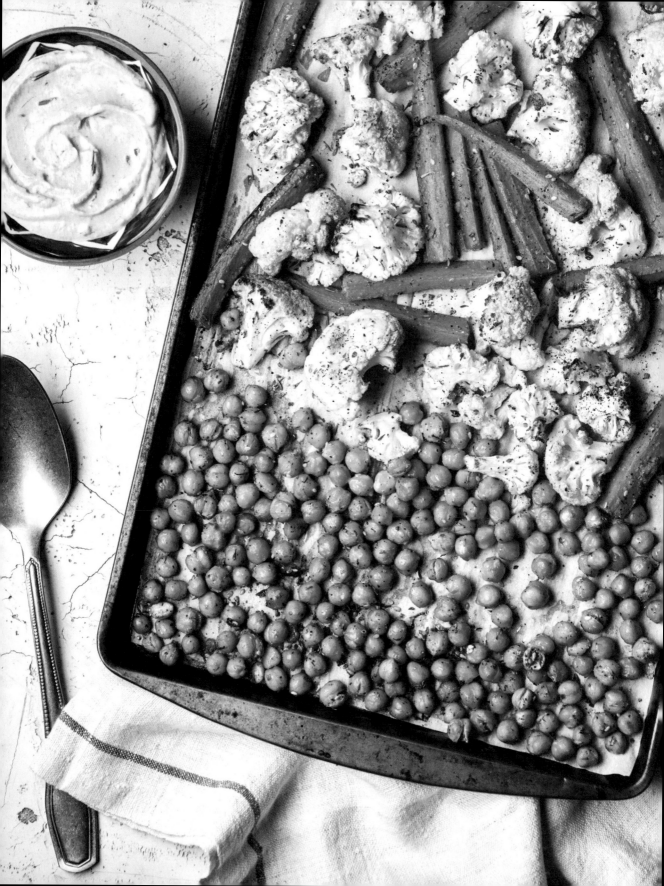

CHAPTER 6

VEGETARIAN MAINS

The Mediterranean diet isn't an inherently vegetarian diet, but because plant foods have so many health benefits, including being linked with a longer, healthier life, it's a very plant-forward diet. That means that vegetarian foods should make up the majority of your plate, and if you want to skip the meat or fish in some of your meals, that's great too.

Plant foods include not only fruits and vegetables, but also beans and other legumes, nuts, seeds, whole grains, and all herbs and spices. Vegetarian meals often include some dairy or eggs too. Even without meat, poultry, or fish, meals can still be well balanced and include plenty of protein.

< Sheet Pan Roasted Chickpeas and Vegetables with Harissa Yogurt, page 90

SOCCA PAN PIZZA WITH HERBED RICOTTA, FRESH TOMATO, AND BALSAMIC GLAZE

Prep Time: 15 minutes / Cook Time: 15 minutes / Serves 2

30 minutes, gluten-free, vegetarian

Socca is a type of quick-cooking Mediterranean flatbread made from chickpea flour instead of wheat. It's a great choice for a pizza base if you're gluten-free, and it's much higher in fiber compared to flatbread or pizza dough made from wheat. Traditionally socca has no leavener and doesn't rise like a typical flatbread, but I have added some baking powder to give this version a lighter texture. Bake this in a large cast-iron or nonstick skillet.

1 cup chickpea flour

1 teaspoon baking powder

½ teaspoon salt

½ teaspoon garlic powder

½ teaspoon onion powder

1½ teaspoons Italian seasoning herb mix, divided

2 tablespoons grated Parmesan cheese

Up to 1 cup warm water

Olive oil, enough to coat the bottom of a skillet

½ cup ricotta cheese

1 ripe tomato, thinly sliced

Balsamic glaze (see Strawberry Caprese Skewers, page 47)

1. Preheat the oven to 425°F and set the rack to the middle position.

2. While the oven is heating, combine the chickpea flour, baking powder, salt, garlic powder, onion powder, 1 teaspoon of the Italian seasoning herb mix, and the Parmesan cheese in a medium bowl.

3. Add most of the water and whisk to combine. The batter should be a pourable consistency like pancake batter, but not as thin as a crepe batter. You may not need all of the water.

4. Heat a large (10- to 12-inch) nonstick or cast-iron skillet on the stovetop over medium-high heat and add the oil.

5. When the pan is hot, pour the batter into the pan and let it cook for a minute, until bubbles start to form. Transfer the pan to the oven and let it cook for 10 minutes, or until the batter starts to turn golden around the edges and looks set.

6. In a small bowl, combine the ricotta cheese and the remaining ½ teaspoon of Italian seasoning herb mix.

7. Remove the pan from the oven and gently spread the ricotta over the crust. Top with the sliced tomatoes and return to the oven for another 2 minutes to let the cheese melt.

8. Use a spatula to remove the dough from the pan. Drizzle it with balsamic glaze, slice, and serve.

INGREDIENT TIP: If you have trouble finding chickpea (also known as garbanzo bean) flour at your regular grocery store, try Whole Foods or a natural foods store or order it online from Bob's Red Mill.

Per Serving: Calories: 318; Total fat: 10g; Total carbs: 37g; Fiber: 6g; Sugar: 9g; Protein: 20g; Sodium: 758mg; Cholesterol: 24mg

CAPRESE-STUFFED PORTOBELLOS

Prep Time: 15 minutes / Cook Time: 30 minutes / Serves 2

gluten-free, vegetarian

Portobello mushrooms are a great meat substitute because they have a hearty, meat-like texture and a rich, meaty umami flavor. Umami has been identified as the fifth taste—after sweet, salty, sour, and bitter—and means "pleasant savory taste" in Japanese. Other umami-rich foods include Parmesan cheese, ripe tomatoes, and fish, which is one reason Mediterranean cooking is so flavorful!

1 tablespoon olive oil, plus extra for drizzling

½ pint cherry or grape tomatoes

¼ teaspoon salt

Pinch freshly ground black pepper

3 medium garlic cloves, minced

4 to 5 large fresh basil leaves, thinly sliced, divided

2 large portobello mushrooms, stems removed

4 pieces mini mozzarella balls (ciliegine), halved

1 tablespoon grated Parmesan cheese

1. Preheat the oven to 350°F.

2. Heat 1 tablespoon of the olive oil in a sauté pan over medium-high heat. Add the tomatoes, salt, and pepper. Pierce a few of the tomatoes as they cook so they give off some juice. Cover and let the tomatoes soften for about 10 minutes.

3. When the tomatoes are mostly softened and begin to break down, add the minced garlic and most of the basil—reserve about 2 teaspoons of basil to garnish at the end. Cook for 30 seconds and then remove from the heat.

4. Oil a baking pan and place the mushrooms gill-side up. If desired, season with salt and pepper.

5. Divide the tomato mixture and the mozzarella balls between the mushrooms. Sprinkle the grated Parmesan cheese evenly over each and, if desired, drizzle the mushrooms with olive oil.

6. Bake them for 20 minutes, or until the mushrooms are softened. If desired, place them under the broiler to brown the cheese a bit. Garnish with the remaining fresh basil.

PREP TIP: This recipe doubles easily, and leftovers are great for lunch or tomorrow's dinner.

Per Serving: Calories: 281; Total fat: 22g; Total carbs: 11g; Fiber: 2g; Sugar: 5g; Protein: 14g; Sodium: 359mg; Cholesterol: 43mg

MUSHROOM-LEEK TORTILLA DE PATATAS

Prep Time: 30 minutes / Cook Time: 50 minutes, plus 5 minutes to rest / Serves 2
gluten-free, vegetarian

Don't let the word tortilla fool you—there's no corn or refried beans here. In Spain, a tortilla de patatas is an omelet with potatoes. It's often served as a tapa—a small portion of food eaten as a snack or appetizer with drinks. This version is packed with flavor, and it's perfect for a light meal or even brunch. Serve it with a Simple Insalata Mista (page 58), or tomato slices drizzled with olive oil and a sprinkle of salt.

1 tablespoon olive oil

1 cup thinly sliced leeks (from 1 leek, light green part only)

4 ounces baby bella (cremini) mushrooms, stemmed and sliced (about 1 cup)

1 small potato, peeled, sliced ¼-inch thick

5 large eggs, beaten

½ cup milk

1 teaspoon Dijon mustard

½ teaspoon dried thyme

½ teaspoon salt

Pinch freshly ground black pepper

3 ounces Gruyère cheese, shredded

1. Preheat the oven to 350°F and set the rack to the middle position.

2. Heat the olive oil in a large sauté pan (nonstick is best) over medium-high heat. Add the leeks, mushrooms, and potato slices and sauté until the leeks are golden and the potatoes start to brown, about 10 minutes.

3. Reduce the heat to medium-low, cover the pan, and let the vegetables cook for another 10 minutes, or until the potatoes begin to soften. If the potato slices stick to the bottom of the pan, add 1 to 2 tablespoons of water to the pan, but be careful because it may splatter.

4. While the vegetables are cooking, combine the beaten eggs, milk, mustard, thyme, salt, pepper, and cheese in a medium bowl and whisk everything together.

5. When the potatoes are soft enough to pierce with a fork or knife, turn off the heat.

6. Transfer the cooked vegetables to an oiled 8-inch oven-safe pan (nonstick is best) and arrange them in a nice layer along the bottom and slightly up the sides of the pan. Alternatively, you can use a glass pie or quiche dish. A smaller pan will give you a nice, tall, moist omelet.

7. Pour the egg mixture over the vegetables and give it a light shake or tap to distribute the eggs evenly through the vegetables.

8. Bake the tortilla for 25 to 30 minutes, or until the eggs are set and the top is golden and puffed. Remove it from the oven, and let it sit for 5 minutes before cutting into it.

SUBSTITUTION TIP: Thin-sliced onion can be substituted for leeks.

VARIATION TIP: This can be eaten hot, warm, or cold, and any leftovers are great for breakfast or lunch.

Per Serving: Calories: 540; Total fat: 33g; Total carbs: 31g; Fiber: 4g; Sugar: 8g; Protein: 33g; Sodium: 913mg; Cholesterol: 509mg

GNOCCHI WITH CREAMY BUTTERNUT SQUASH AND BLUE CHEESE SAUCE

Prep Time: 10 minutes / Cook Time: 20 minutes / Serves 2

30 minutes, vegetarian

This is grown-up mac and cheese that you could easily serve to company. Of course, it's wonderful that butternut squash is packed with beta-carotene, but it's also a pretty amazing substitute for lots of cream and cheese when making mac and cheese. I personally love a little bit of Gorgonzola Dolce (a mild, slightly sweet Italian blue cheese) here, but a sharp cheddar or smoked Gouda would also be great.

5 ounces frozen diced butternut squash

¼ cup low-sodium vegetable stock

Pinch salt

Pinch nutmeg

Pinch cayenne pepper

Pinch freshly ground black pepper

8 ounces prepared, packaged gnocchi

1 tablespoon olive oil

1 garlic clove, minced

2 fresh sage leaves

1 ounce Gorgonzola Dolce or other mild blue cheese

1 tablespoon heavy cream (optional)

1. In a saucepan, bring the butternut squash and vegetable stock to a boil. Cover, and reduce the heat to medium-low. Simmer for 10 minutes, or until the squash is very tender.

2. Transfer the squash and vegetable stock to a blender. Add the salt, nutmeg, cayenne, and black pepper, and blend on low speed until it's completely smooth. (Make sure your blender is no more than half full or the hot liquid may erupt through the lid.)

3. Taste and add additional salt if needed. Set the squash aside.

4. Using the same saucepan, cook the gnocchi according to package directions.

5. While the gnocchi cooks, heat the olive oil in a large sauté pan over medium-high heat. Add the garlic and sage and sauté for 45 seconds, just until the garlic and sage are fragrant.

6. Carefully add the puréed squash to the sauté pan. Stir in the cheese and cream, if using.

7. Add the cooked gnocchi to the pan and gently stir to coat with the sauce. Taste and add any salt, pepper, or another pinch of nutmeg as needed. Remove the sage leaves before serving.

PREP TIP: Gnocchi are made from potato and flour and they cook very quickly. Make sure you remove them from the heat as soon as the gnocchi float to the top of the pan. I like to use a slotted spoon and scoop them right from the water and into the sauce.

SUBSTITUTION TIP: Experiment with different types of cheese, like sharp cheddar, smoked Gouda, or Gruyère. You may need a bit more than the 2 ounces called for in the recipe because these are all milder in flavor than blue cheese.

Per Serving: Calories: 653; Total fat: 23g; Total carbs: 100g; Fiber: 2g; Sugar: 0g; Protein: 17g; Sodium: 1016mg; Cholesterol: 21mg

ROASTED RATATOUILLE PASTA

Prep Time: 10 minutes / Cook Time: 20 minutes / Serves 2

30 minutes, dairy-free, vegan, vegetarian

Traditional ratatouille is a vegetable stew from southern France. It features fresh eggplant, sweet peppers, zucchini, tomatoes, and whatever else is in season. I love roasting or grilling these same vegetables because the higher heat caramelizes the sugars in the sweeter vegetables and brings out the natural smokiness in the eggplant and zucchini. Serve this dish warm for dinner or make it ahead of time and eat it at room temperature or cold as a picnic salad.

1 small eggplant (about 8 ounces)

1 small zucchini

1 portobello mushroom

1 Roma tomato, halved

½ medium sweet red pepper, seeded

½ teaspoon salt, plus additional for the pasta water

1 teaspoon Italian herb seasoning

1 tablespoon olive oil

2 cups farfalle pasta (about 8 ounces)

2 tablespoons minced sun-dried tomatoes in olive oil with herbs

2 tablespoons prepared pesto

1. Slice the ends off the eggplant and zucchini. Cut them lengthwise into ½-inch slices.

2. Place the eggplant, zucchini, mushroom, tomato, and red pepper in a large bowl and sprinkle with ½ teaspoon of salt. Using your hands, toss the vegetables well so that they're covered evenly with the salt. Let them rest for about 10 minutes.

3. While the vegetables are resting, preheat the oven to 400°F and set the rack to the bottom position. Line a baking sheet with parchment paper.

4. When the oven is hot, drain off any liquid from the vegetables and pat them dry with a paper towel. Add the Italian herb seasoning and olive oil to the vegetables and toss well to coat both sides.

5. Lay the vegetables out in a single layer on the baking sheet. Roast them for 15 to 20 minutes, flipping them over after about 10 minutes or once they start to brown on the underside. When the vegetables are charred in spots, remove them from the oven.

6. While the vegetables are roasting, fill a large saucepan with water. Add salt and cook the pasta according to package directions. Drain the pasta, reserving ½ cup of the pasta water.

7. When cool enough to handle, cut the vegetables into large chunks (about 2 inches) and add them to the hot pasta.

8. Stir in the sun-dried tomatoes and pesto and toss everything well.

PREP TIP: If it's too hot to turn on the oven, grill the vegetables instead of roasting them.

Per Serving: Calories: 612; Total fat: 16g; Total carbs: 110g; Fiber: 23g; Sugar: 16g; Protein: 23g; Sodium: 776mg; Cholesterol: 2mg

MUSHROOM RAGÙ WITH PARMESAN POLENTA

Prep Time: 20 minutes / Cook Time: 30 minutes / Serves 2

vegetarian

Mushrooms have such a nice meaty texture and umami flavor, they're every bit as satisfying as meat in this recipe. Whenever I cook soups, stews, or any other dish with mushrooms, I use a mix of baby bellas and a small handful of dried mushrooms. Porcinis are my favorite for their rich flavor.

½ ounce dried porcini mushrooms (optional but recommended)

2 tablespoons olive oil

1 pound baby bella (cremini) mushrooms, quartered

1 large shallot, minced (about ⅓ cup)

1 garlic clove, minced

1 tablespoon flour

2 teaspoons tomato paste

½ cup red wine

1 cup mushroom stock (or reserved liquid from soaking the porcini mushrooms, if using)

½ teaspoon dried thyme

1 fresh rosemary sprig

1½ cups water

½ teaspoon salt

⅓ cup instant polenta

2 tablespoons grated Parmesan cheese

1. If using the dried porcini mushrooms, soak them in 1 cup of hot water for about 15 minutes to soften them. When they're softened, scoop them out of the water, reserving the soaking liquid. (I strain it through a coffee filter to remove any possible grit.) Mince the porcini mushrooms.

2. Heat the olive oil in a large sauté pan over medium-high heat. Add the mushrooms, shallot, and garlic, and sauté for 10 minutes, or until the vegetables are wilted and starting to caramelize.

3. Add the flour and tomato paste, and cook for another 30 seconds. Add the red wine, mushroom stock or porcini soaking liquid, thyme, and rosemary. Bring the mixture to a boil, stirring constantly until it thickens. Reduce the heat and let it simmer for 10 minutes.

4. While the mushrooms are simmering, bring the water to a boil in a saucepan and add salt.

5. Add the instant polenta and stir quickly while it thickens. Stir in the Parmesan cheese. Taste and add additional salt if needed.

INGREDIENT TIP: Make sure you buy instant polenta, which cooks in seconds. Regular polenta takes about 45 minutes to cook.

INGREDIENT TIP: The website Nuts.com is a great source for dried mushrooms (and nuts, of course!).

Per Serving: Calories: 451; Total fat: 16g; Total carbs: 58g; Fiber: 5g; Sugar: 6g; Protein: 14g; Sodium: 165mg; Cholesterol: 5mg

BEET AND CARROT FRITTERS WITH YOGURT SAUCE

Prep Time: 15 minutes / Cook Time: 15 minutes / Serves 2

30 minutes, gluten-free, vegetarian

It's so easy to "eat the rainbow" with this recipe. I love the gorgeous colors in these fritters from the combination of beets and carrots with a little bit of scallion and parsley thrown in. Beets have unique phytocompounds called betalains. They have antioxidant, anti-inflammatory, and detoxification powers, and they're especially protective against heart disease and cancer.

For the yogurt sauce

⅓ cup plain Greek yogurt

1 tablespoon freshly squeezed lemon juice

Zest of ½ lemon

¼ teaspoon garlic powder

¼ teaspoon salt

For the fritters

1 large carrot, peeled

1 small potato, peeled

1 medium golden or red beet, peeled

1 scallion, minced

2 tablespoons fresh minced parsley

¼ cup brown rice flour or unseasoned bread crumbs

¼ teaspoon garlic powder

¼ teaspoon salt

1 large egg, beaten

¼ cup feta cheese, crumbled

2 tablespoons olive oil (more if needed)

To make the yogurt sauce

In a small bowl, mix together the yogurt, lemon juice and zest, garlic powder, and salt. Set aside.

To make the fritters

1. Shred the carrot, potato, and beet in a food processor with the shredding blade. You can also use a mandoline with a julienne shredding blade or a vegetable peeler. Squeeze out any moisture from the vegetables and place them in a large bowl.

2. Add the scallion, parsley, rice flour, garlic powder, salt, and egg. Stir the mixture well to combine. Add the feta cheese and stir briefly, leaving chunks of feta cheese throughout.

3. Heat a large nonstick sauté pan over medium-high heat and add 1 tablespoon of the olive oil.

4. Make the fritters by scooping about 3 tablespoons of the vegetable mixture into your hands and flattening it into a firm disc about 3 inches in diameter.

5. Place 2 fritters at a time in the pan and let them cook for about two minutes. Check to see if the underside is golden, and then flip and repeat on the other side. Remove from the heat, add the rest of the olive oil to the pan, and repeat with the remaining vegetable mixture.

6. To serve, spoon about 1 tablespoon of the yogurt sauce on top of each fritter.

INGREDIENT TIP: If you like to make vegetable fritters, brown rice flour is a nice ingredient to keep on hand, because it gives the fritters a nice, crispy crunch. If you don't have it, unseasoned bread crumbs can easily be substituted.

VARIATION TIP: Try this with any kind of shredded vegetables. Zucchini, sweet potato, parsnip, or butternut squash would all work. (If using zucchini, press it to remove additional moisture.)

Per Serving: Calories: 295; Total fat: 14g; Total carbs: 44g; Fiber: 5g; Sugar: 11g; Protein: 6g; Sodium: 482; Cholesterol: 74mg

MOROCCAN-INSPIRED CHICKPEA TAGINE

Prep Time: 20 minutes / Cook Time: 40 minutes / Serves 2, with leftovers for lunch

dairy-free, gluten-free, vegan, vegetarian

A tagine is a cone-shaped earthenware pot that's used to cook a Moroccan stew also called tagine. Luckily, a Dutch oven works just as well for this stew. Moroccan dishes are known for their aromatic spices, which often include both sweet spices like cinnamon and savory or hot spices like cumin and harissa. Tagines are packed with health benefits not only from the vegetables, but also from those antioxidant-packed spices.

2 tablespoons olive oil

½ onion, diced

1 garlic clove, minced

2 cups cauliflower florets

1 cup diced eggplant (large dice)

1 medium carrot, cut into 1-inch pieces

2 small red potatoes, cut into 1-inch pieces

1 (28-ounce) can whole tomatoes with their juices

1 (15-ounce) can chickpeas, drained and rinsed

1 cup water

1 teaspoon sugar

1 teaspoon cumin

½ teaspoon turmeric

½ teaspoon cinnamon

½ teaspoon salt

1 to 2 teaspoons harissa paste

1. Heat the olive oil in a Dutch oven over medium-high heat. Add the onion and sauté for 5 minutes.

2. Add the garlic, cauliflower, eggplant, carrot, potatoes, and tomatoes. Stir, breaking up the tomatoes with a spatula. Add the chickpeas, water, sugar, cumin, turmeric, cinnamon, and salt.

3. Bring the mixture to a boil, and then reduce the heat to medium-low. Add 1 teaspoon of the harissa. Taste and add another 1 teaspoon if you prefer the stew spicier.

4. Cover the pot and let the stew simmer for about 40 minutes, or until the vegetables are tender. Taste and add additional salt and any other spices, if needed.

Per Serving: Calories: 294; Total fat: 10g; Total carbs: 46g; Fiber: 12g; Sugar: 13g; Protein: 11g; Sodium: 338mg; Cholesterol: 0mg

STUFFED PEPPER STEW

Prep Time: 20 minutes / Cook Time: 50 minutes / Serves 2, with leftovers for lunch
dairy-free, gluten-free, vegan, vegetarian

Lentils are packed with protein and fiber, and along with other legumes, are an important part of the Mediterranean diet. All legumes have wonderful health benefits: When eaten regularly, they can reduce your cholesterol, stabilize your blood sugar, and even help you lose weight. They're a great stand-in for ground beef in this recipe, which is like stuffed peppers in a bowl.

2 tablespoons olive oil

2 sweet peppers, diced (about 2 cups)

½ large onion, minced

1 garlic clove, minced

1 teaspoon oregano

1 tablespoon gluten-free vegetarian Worcestershire sauce

1 cup low-sodium vegetable stock

1 cup low-sodium tomato juice

¼ cup brown lentils

¼ cup brown rice

Salt

1. Heat olive oil in a Dutch oven over medium-high heat. Add the sweet peppers and onion and sauté for 10 minutes, or until the peppers are wilted and the onion starts to turn golden.

2. Add the garlic, oregano, and Worcestershire sauce, and cook for another 30 seconds. Add the vegetable stock, tomato juice, lentils, and rice.

3. Bring the mixture to a boil. Cover, and reduce the heat to medium-low. Simmer for 45 minutes, or until the rice is cooked and the lentils are softened. Season with salt.

SUBSTITUTION TIP: If you prefer to use meat instead of lentils, try lean ground beef, turkey, or lamb, and beef stock instead of vegetable stock.

PREP TIP: If the stew seems too thick, add water or extra stock to thin it out.

Per Serving: Calories: 379; Total fat: 16g; Total carbs: 53g; Fiber: 7g; Sugar: 14g; Protein: 11g; Sodium: 392mg; Cholesterol: 0mg

ONE-PAN MUSHROOM PASTA WITH MASCARPONE

Prep Time: 10 minutes / Cook Time: 20 minutes / Serves 2

30 minutes, vegetarian

Is there anything better than a one-pan meal that's on the table in about 30 minutes? I think not! This pasta dish is a luscious treat because of the addition of just a little bit of mascarpone cheese at the end. It reminds me of so many amazing pasta dishes I had in Italy. If you're limiting saturated fat, feel free to skip the mascarpone. It's still delicious without it.

2 tablespoons olive oil

1 large shallot, minced

8 ounces baby bella (cremini) mushrooms, sliced

¼ cup dry sherry

1 teaspoon dried thyme

2 cups low-sodium vegetable stock

6 ounces dry pappardelle pasta

2 tablespoons mascarpone cheese

Salt

Freshly ground black pepper

1. Heat olive oil in a large sauté pan over medium-high heat. Add the shallot and mushrooms and sauté for 10 minutes, or until the mushrooms have given up much of their liquid.

2. Add the sherry, thyme, and vegetable stock. Bring the mixture to a boil.

3. Add the pasta, breaking it up as needed so it fits into the pan and is covered by the liquid. Return the mixture to a boil. Cover, and reduce the heat to medium-low. Let the pasta cook for 10 minutes, or until al dente. Stir it occasionally so it doesn't stick. If the sauce gets too dry, add some water or additional chicken stock.

4. When the pasta is tender, stir in the mascarpone cheese and season with salt and pepper.

5. The sauce will thicken up a bit when it's off the heat.

VARIATION TIP: Try adding some baby spinach to the pan at the end. Just stir it in and let it wilt for a few seconds.

PREP TIP: Most dried pasta comes in either an 8-ounce or 16-ounce package. If you use all 8 ounces, you may not have enough sauce. A kitchen scale can be very helpful for one-pan pasta dishes and also for weighing out proteins, to avoid waste.

Per Serving: Calories: 517; Total fat: 18g; Total carbs: 69g; Fiber: 3g; Sugar: 2g; Protein: 16g; Sodium: 141mg; Cholesterol: 20mg

LENTIL BOLOGNESE

Prep Time: 15 minutes / Cook Time: 50 minutes, plus time to cook the lentils / Serves 2, with leftovers for lunch

gluten-free, vegetarian

Traditional Bolognese sauce is made with meat, sautéed vegetables, and a tomato sauce. Swapping in lentils for the meat still provides the protein and heartiness of the sauce, while also adding nutrients such as fiber.

½ large onion

1 medium celery stalk

1 large carrot

1 garlic clove

2 tablespoons olive oil

1 (28-ounce) can crushed tomatoes

1 cup red wine

½ teaspoon sugar

½ teaspoon salt

1 cup cooked lentils (prepared from ½ cup dry)

2 tablespoons cream

1. Place the onion, celery, carrot, and garlic in a food processor and pulse until the vegetables are finely minced.

2. Heat the olive oil in a Dutch oven over medium-high heat. Add the minced vegetable mixture and sauté for 10 minutes, or until the vegetables are wilted.

3. Add the tomatoes, wine, sugar, and salt. Bring the sauce to a boil. Cover the pot and reduce the heat to medium-low. Let the sauce simmer for 30 minutes, or until the vegetables are tender.

4. Add the cooked lentils and the cream. Cook for another 5 minutes and season with additional salt, if needed.

VARIATION TIP: To make this vegan, omit the cream.

SUBSTITUTION TIP: 1 cup of minced mushrooms or cooked bulgur wheat can be substituted for the lentils.

Per Serving: Calories: 269; Total fat: 8g; Total carbs: 32g; Fiber: 16g; Sugar: 15g; Protein: 10g; Sodium: 308mg; Cholesterol: 1mg

ORZO-STUFFED TOMATOES

Prep Time: 15 minutes / Cook Time: 30 minutes / Serves 2

dairy-free, vegetarian

Whenever I cook grains or small pasta like orzo or couscous, I try to make extra to use in another meal. Most will freeze very nicely, and if you lay them out on a baking pan to cool, they won't stick together as much in the freezer. Just scoop out the portion needed for your next recipe. This recipe calls for less than 1 cup of cooked orzo, but the grain makes it more of a light meal. It can be served hot or chilled.

1 tablespoon olive oil

1 small zucchini, minced

½ medium onion, minced

1 garlic clove, minced

⅔ cup cooked orzo (from ¼ cup dry orzo, cooked according to package instructions, or precooked)

½ teaspoon salt

2 teaspoons dried oregano

6 medium round tomatoes (not Roma)

1. Preheat the oven to 350°F.

2. Heat the olive oil in a large sauté pan over medium-high heat. Add the zucchini, onion, and garlic and sauté for 15 minutes, or until the vegetables turn golden.

3. Add the orzo, salt, and oregano and stir to heat through. Remove the pan from the heat and set aside.

4. Cut about ½ inch from the top of each tomato. With a paring knife, cut around the inner core of the tomato to remove about half of the flesh. Reserve for another recipe or a salad.

5. Stuff each tomato with the orzo mixture.

6. If serving hot, put the tomatoes in a baking dish, or, if they'll fit, a muffin tin. Roast the tomatoes for about 15 minutes, or until they're soft. Don't overcook them or they won't hold together. If desired, this can also be served without roasting the tomatoes.

SUBSTITUTION TIP: Instead of zucchini, try roasted or raw sweet peppers or summer squash. You can also substitute any other small grain (quinoa, bulgur, or sorghum) for the orzo.

Per Serving: Calories: 241; Total fat: 8g; Total carbs: 38g; Fiber: 6g; Sugar: 11g; Protein: 7g; Sodium: 301mg; Cholesterol: 0mg

GRILLED EGGPLANT STACKS

Prep Time: 20 minutes / Cook Time: 10 minutes / Serves 2

30 minutes, gluten-free, vegetarian

Eggplant is thought to have its roots in Africa or Asia, although it's most often associated with Italian cooking and eggplant Parmesan. This recipe is a lightened-up version of traditional eggplant Parmesan, and I love to make it on the grill because the high heat really brings out a tasty smokiness from eggplant. To remove any bitterness, make sure you salt your eggplant generously and let it sit for about 15 minutes before you cook it.

1 medium eggplant, cut crosswise into 8 slices

¼ teaspoon salt

1 teaspoon Italian herb seasoning mix

2 tablespoons olive oil

1 large tomato, cut into 4 slices

4 (1-ounce) slices of buffalo mozzarella

Fresh basil, for garnish

1. Place the eggplant slices in a colander set in the sink or over a bowl. Sprinkle both sides with the salt. Let the eggplant sit for 15 minutes.

2. While the eggplant is resting, heat the grill to medium-high heat (about 350°F).

3. Pat the eggplant dry with paper towels and place it in a mixing bowl. Sprinkle it with the Italian herb seasoning mix and olive oil. Toss well to coat.

4. Grill the eggplant for 5 minutes, or until it has grill marks and is lightly charred. Flip each eggplant slice over, and grill on the second side for another 5 minutes.

5. Flip the eggplant slices back over and top four of the slices with a slice of tomato and a slice of mozzarella. Top each stack with one of the remaining four slices of eggplant.

6. Turn the grill down to low and cover it to let the cheese melt. Check after 30 seconds and remove when the cheese is soft and mostly melted.

7. Sprinkle with fresh basil slices.

PREP TIP: Eggplant contains at least 90 percent water and really reduces in thickness when it's grilled, so make sure you cut your slices at least 1 inch thick.

Per Serving: Calories: 354; Total fat: 29g; Total carbs: 19g; Fiber: 9g; Sugar: 9g; Protein: 13g; Sodium: 340mg; Cholesterol: 40mg

ASPARAGUS AND MUSHROOM FARROTTO

Prep Time: 20 minutes / Cook Time: 45 minutes / Serves 2

Porcini mushroom risotto is one of my favorite comfort foods. It's rich, creamy, and packed with flavor. When I discovered I could use whole-grain farro as a stand-in for starchy arborio rice, I was sold! Farro is a Mediterranean ancient grain that's higher in fiber and has a lower glycemic index. Now porcini "farrotto" is my new favorite comfort food. Risotto (or farrotto) should cook slowly, and it's important to keep a close eye on it, stir frequently, and add more liquid as it cooks.

½ ounce dried
porcini mushrooms

1 cup hot water

3 cups low-sodium
vegetable stock

2 tablespoons olive oil

½ large onion, minced
(about 1 cup)

1 garlic clove

1 cup diced mushrooms
(about 4 ounces)

¾ cup farro

½ cup dry white wine

½ teaspoon dried thyme

4 ounces asparagus,
cut into ½-inch pieces
(about 1 cup)

2 tablespoons grated
Parmesan cheese

Salt

1. Soak the dried mushrooms in the hot water for about 15 minutes. When they're softened, drain the mushrooms, reserving the liquid. (I like to strain the liquid through a coffee filter in case there's any grit.) Mince the porcini mushrooms.

2. Add the mushroom liquid and vegetable stock to a medium saucepan and bring it to a boil. Reduce the heat to low just to keep it warm.

3. Heat the olive oil in a Dutch oven over high heat. Add the onion, garlic, and mushrooms, and sauté for 10 minutes.

4. Add the farro to the Dutch oven and sauté it for 3 minutes to toast.

5. Add the wine, thyme, and one ladleful of the hot mushroom and chicken stock. Bring it to a boil while stirring the farro. Do not cover the pot while the farro is cooking.

6. Reduce the heat to medium. When the liquid is absorbed, add another ladleful or two at a time to the pot, stirring occasionally, until the farro is cooked through. Keep an eye on the heat, to make sure it doesn't cook too quickly.

7. When the farro is al dente, add the asparagus and another ladleful of stock. Cook for another 3 to 5 minutes, or until the asparagus is softened.

8. Stir in Parmesan cheese and season with salt.

VARIATION TIP: You can make this dish with any combination of vegetables you like, or add leftover shredded chicken to the mix.

Per Serving: Calories: 341; Total fat: 16g; Total carbs: 26g; Fiber: 5g; Sugar: 4g; Protein: 13g; Sodium: 259mg; Cholesterol: 5mg

SHEET PAN ROASTED CHICKPEAS AND VEGETABLES WITH HARISSA YOGURT

Prep Time: 10 minutes / Cook Time: 30 minutes / Serves 2

gluten-free, vegan, vegetarian

When your schedule gets busy, back-pocket meals can be a lifesaver. They're the kind of meals that don't need a recipe, require minimal prep time, and come together quickly because you usually have the ingredients on hand. Vegetarian meals like this one make the best back-pocket meals because there's no thawing or cooking of meat. Instead, the chickpeas and yogurt provide the protein.

4 cups cauliflower florets (about ½ small head)

2 medium carrots, peeled, halved, and then sliced into quarters lengthwise

2 tablespoons olive oil, divided

½ teaspoon garlic powder, divided

½ teaspoon salt, divided

2 teaspoons za'atar spice mix, divided

1 (15-ounce) can chickpeas, drained, rinsed, and patted dry

¾ cup plain Greek yogurt

1 teaspoon harissa spice paste

1. Preheat the oven to 400°F and set the rack to the middle position. Line a sheet pan with foil or parchment paper.

2. Place the cauliflower and carrots in a large bowl. Drizzle with 1 tablespoon olive oil and sprinkle with ¼ teaspoon of garlic powder, ¼ teaspoon of salt, and 1 teaspoon of za'atar. Toss well to combine.

3. Spread the vegetables onto one half of the sheet pan in a single layer.

4. Place the chickpeas in the same bowl and season with the remaining 1 tablespoon of oil, ¼ teaspoon of garlic powder, and ¼ teaspoon of salt, and the remaining za'atar. Toss well to combine.

5. Spread the chickpeas onto the other half of the sheet pan.

6. Roast for 30 minutes, or until the vegetables are tender and the chickpeas start to turn golden. Flip the vegetables halfway through the cooking time, and give the chickpeas a stir so they cook evenly.

7. The chickpeas may need an extra few minutes if you like them crispy. If so, remove the vegetables and leave the chickpeas in until they're cooked to desired crispiness.

8. While the vegetables are roasting, combine the yogurt and harissa in a small bowl. Taste, and add additional harissa as desired.

INGREDIENT TIP: Za'atar is a classic Middle Eastern spice blend that's typically made from sesame seeds, marjoram, sumac, oregano, and thyme—although the spice combination can vary. Harissa is a Tunisian spiced hot chili sauce. Look for them in the spice section of your grocery store or order them online.

Per Serving: Calories: 467; Total fat: 23g; Total carbs: 54g; Fiber: 15g; Sugar: 18g; Protein: 18g; Sodium: 632mg; Cholesterol: 19mg

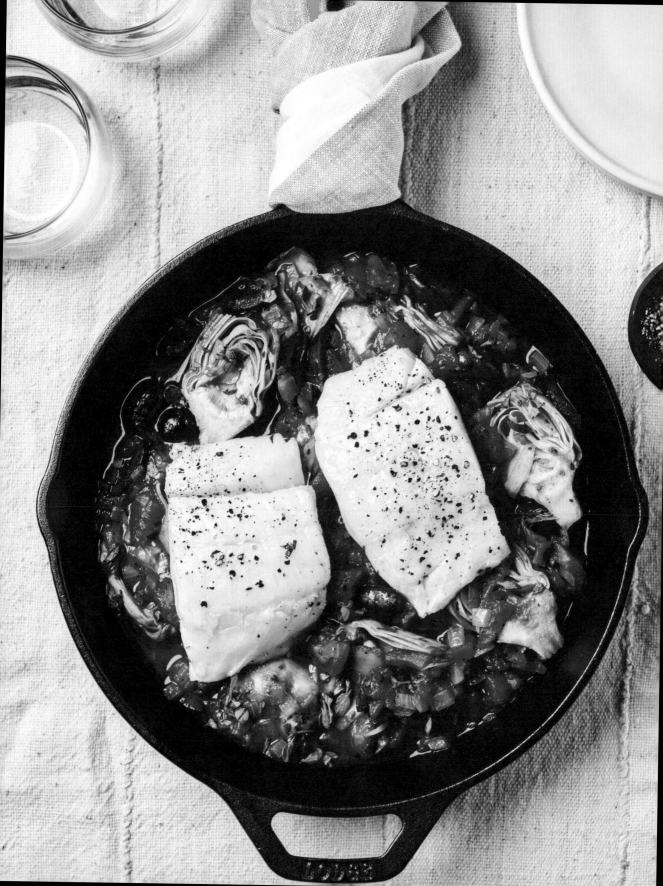

CHAPTER 7

FISH AND SEAFOOD MAINS

Seafood is an important part of the Mediterranean diet. Traditionally, people in the countries bordering the Mediterranean Sea eat far more fish than meat or poultry, and it's one of the reasons they have lower rates of heart disease. Seafood is a lean and healthy source of protein, and fish that have more fat—such as salmon, sardines, anchovies, and mackerel—are rich in omega-3 fatty acids.

Eating more fish is linked with a lower risk of heart disease, metabolic diseases, and even depression, likely because of those omega-3 fatty acids. The Mediterranean diet food pyramid recommends eating seafood at least twice each week.

Although this diet emphasizes using fresh ingredients, some fish—such as sardines, anchovies, and mackerel—are more readily available canned than fresh. These are actually great options to stock in your pantry. They're still packed with those good fats, but since they're already cooked and portioned, they're great time-savers.

An excellent resource to identify sustainable seafood options at the grocery store is seafoodwatch.org, the website of the Monterey Bay Aquarium Seafood Watch Program. This information is also available in the Seafood Watch app.

< Pan Roasted Wild Cod with Tomatoes, Olives, and Artichokes, page 104

PISTACHIO-CRUSTED WHITEFISH

Prep Time: 10 minutes / Cook Time: 20 minutes / Serves 2

30 minutes

Whitefish is a general term for any lean, quick-cooking, white-colored fish like cod, haddock, pollock, or flounder. While lower in omega-3s than salmon or other fatty fish, whitefish is still a great source of protein and counts toward the recommended two weekly servings of seafood. If there are several options, ask your fishmonger what's freshest and what they recommend.

¼ **cup shelled pistachios**

1 tablespoon
fresh parsley

1 tablespoon grated
Parmesan cheese

1 tablespoon panko
bread crumbs

2 tablespoons olive oil

¼ teaspoon salt

10 ounces skinless
**whitefish (1 large piece or
2 smaller ones)**

1. Preheat the oven to 350°F and set the rack to the middle position. Line a sheet pan with foil or parchment paper.

2. Combine all of the ingredients except the fish in a mini food processor, and pulse until the nuts are finely ground. Alternatively, you can mince the nuts with a chef's knife and combine the ingredients by hand in a small bowl.

3. Place the fish on the sheet pan. Spread the nut mixture evenly over the fish and pat it down lightly.

4. Bake the fish for 20 to 30 minutes, depending on the thickness, until it flakes easily with a fork.

PREP TIP: Keep in mind that a thicker cut of fish takes a bit longer to bake. You'll know it's done when it's opaque, flakes apart easily with a fork, or reaches an internal temperature of 145°F.

SUBSTITUTION TIP: Panko bread crumbs have a larger, lighter crumb that crisps nicely in the oven, but you can also substitute plain or Italian-seasoned bread crumbs.

Per Serving: Calories: 267; Total fat: 18g; Total carbs: 1g; Fiber: 0g; Sugar: 0g; Protein: 28g; Sodium: 85mg; Cholesterol: 71mg

WILD COD OREGANATA

Prep Time: 10 minutes / Cook Time: 20 minutes / Serves 2
30 minutes

Wild cod is a mild-tasting, quick-cooking sustainable fish. It's also very low in calories and high in protein. A plain, 5-ounce portion has less than 150 calories and about 30 grams of protein, so it's a great choice to help you maintain a healthy weight.

10 ounces wild cod
(1 large piece or
2 smaller ones)

⅓ cup panko
bread crumbs

1 tablespoon
dried oregano

Zest of 1 lemon

½ teaspoon salt

Pinch freshly ground
black pepper

1 tablespoon olive oil

2 tablespoons freshly
squeezed lemon juice

2 tablespoons white wine

1 tablespoon minced
fresh parsley

1. Preheat the oven to 350°F. Place the cod in a baking dish and pat it dry with a paper towel.

2. In a small bowl, combine the panko, oregano, lemon zest, salt, pepper, and olive oil and mix well. Pat the panko mixture onto the fish.

3. Combine the lemon juice and wine in a small bowl and pour it around the fish.

4. Bake the fish for 20 minutes, or until it flakes apart easily and reaches an internal temperature of 145°F.

5. Garnish with fresh minced parsley.

PREP TIP: Whenever you have a small amount of leftover wine, freeze it in an ice cube tray. It's perfect for recipes like this one that call for a small amount of wine.

Per Serving: Calories: 203; Total fat: 8g; Total carbs: 9g; Fiber: 2g; Sugar: 1g; Protein: 23g; Sodium: 149mg; Cholesterol: 90mg

EASY SHRIMP PAELLA

Prep Time: 20 minutes / Cook Time: 1 hour 5 minutes / Serves 2

Dairy-free, gluten-free

Paella is one of the best-known dishes of Spain. It's named for the pan it's cooked in, and while the base is rice and usually seafood, there are a great many variations of this dish. The beauty of paella is that it's the ultimate one-pan meal that can be sized down for two as it is here or, if you have a full-sized paella pan, a larger batch can easily feed a crowd.

2 tablespoons olive oil

½ large onion, minced

1 garlic clove, minced

4 ounces chorizo sausage, removed from casing

1 cup diced tomato (about 1 medium tomato)

½ teaspoon sweet paprika

Generous pinch saffron

½ cup medium- or short-grain rice

½ cup dry white wine

1¼ cups low-sodium chicken stock

8 ounces large raw shrimp

1 cup frozen peas

¼ cup jarred roasted red peppers, cut into strips (about 1 whole pepper)

Salt

1. Heat the olive oil in a large sauté pan over medium-high heat. Add the onion, garlic, and chorizo, and sauté for 10 minutes, or until the onion is wilted and the chorizo is cooked.

2. Add the tomato, paprika, saffron, and rice, and stir for 3 minutes to toast the rice and spices.

3. Add the wine and chicken stock and stir. Bring the mixture to a boil. Cover and reduce the heat to medium-low, and let the paella cook for 45 minutes, or until the rice is just about tender and most, but not all, of the liquid has been absorbed.

4. Add the shrimp, peas, and roasted red peppers. Cover and cook for another 5 minutes. Season with salt.

SUBSTITUTION TIP: Feel free to use any type of seafood in this recipe. Traditional options include mussels, calamari rings, shrimp or prawns, clams, and lobster.

Per Serving: Calories: 645; Total fat: 27g; Total carbs: 60g; Fiber: 7g; Sugar: 9g; Protein: 42g; Sodium: 686mg; Cholesterol: 262mg

CIOPPINO

Prep Time: 10 minutes / Cook Time: 20 minutes / Serves 2, with leftovers for lunch
30 minutes, dairy-free, gluten-free

Technically, cioppino is from San Francisco, not the Mediterranean, but this hearty seafood stew is a family favorite that's full of so many Mediterranean flavors, I had to include it. This is the kind of meal you have to do a little bit of planning for, so you have the fish available, but once you have the ingredients assembled you can pull it together in minutes—and it's special enough to serve to company. Serve this with rice or with some crusty sourdough bread to scoop up the sauce.

2 tablespoons olive oil

½ green pepper, diced

½ small onion, diced

2 teaspoons dried oregano

2 teaspoons dried basil

½ cup dry white wine

1 (14.5-ounce) can diced tomatoes with basil

1 (8-ounce) can no-salt-added tomato sauce

1 (6.5-ounce) can minced clams with their juice

8 ounces peeled, deveined raw shrimp

4 ounces any whitefish (a thick piece works best)

3 tablespoons fresh parsley

Salt

Freshly ground black pepper

1. Heat the olive oil in a Dutch oven over medium heat. Add the green pepper and onion and sauté for 5 minutes, or until softened.

2. Add the oregano, basil, wine, chopped tomatoes, and tomato sauce. Bring the mixture to a boil. Reduce the heat and simmer for 5 minutes.

3. Add the clams, shrimp, and whitefish, and let the cioppino cook for about 10 minutes, until the fish is opaque and cooked through. The shrimp should be bright pink.

4. Add the fresh parsley. Taste and add salt and freshly ground black pepper to taste.

PREP TIP: The base of this stew can be prepared ahead of time, or even the day before, but don't add the fish until just before serving.

INGREDIENT TIP: If you can't find peeled, deveined shrimp at the fish counter, check the frozen fish section.

Per Serving: Calories: 222; Total fat: 8g; Total carbs: 11g; Fiber: 4g; Sugar: 7g; Protein: 23g; Sodium: 721mg; Cholesterol: 110mg

SEARED SCALLOPS WITH WHITE BEAN PURÉE

Prep Time: 15 minutes / Cook Time: 15 minutes / Serves 2
30 minutes, dairy-free, gluten-free

Scallops always seem like a special, elegant restaurant meal, but they're quick and very easy to prepare. In addition, they're extremely low in calories and high in protein, so even though they taste rich and decadent, they're actually quite lean and healthy. Scallops are also a good source of the antioxidant selenium, and they provide omega-3 fatty acids.

4 tablespoons olive oil, divided

2 garlic cloves

2 teaspoons minced fresh rosemary

1 (15-ounce) can white cannellini beans, drained and rinsed

½ cup low-sodium chicken stock

Salt

Freshly ground black pepper

10 ounces sea scallops (about 6)

1. To make the bean purée, heat 2 tablespoons of olive oil in a saucepan over medium-high heat. Add the garlic and sauté for 30 seconds, or just until it's fragrant. Don't let it burn. Add the rosemary and remove the pan from the heat.

2. Add the white beans and chicken stock to the pan, return it to the heat, and stir. Bring the beans to a boil. Reduce the heat to low and simmer for 5 minutes.

3. Transfer the beans to a blender and purée them for 30 seconds, or until they're smooth. Taste and season with salt and pepper. Let them sit in the blender with the lid on to keep them warm while you prepare the scallops.

4. Pat the scallops dry with a paper towel and season them with salt and pepper.

5. Heat the remaining 2 tablespoons of olive oil in a large sauté pan. When the oil is shimmering, add the scallops, flat-side down.

6. Cook the scallops for 2 minutes, or until they're golden on the bottom. Flip them over and cook for another 1 to 2 minutes, or until opaque and slightly firm.

7. To serve, divide the bean purée between two plates and top with the scallops.

PREP TIP: Scallops cook very quickly, and since they have very little fat they become dry if overcooked. Prepare them just before you're ready to assemble your meal.

Per Serving: Calories: 465; Total fat: 29g; Total carbs: 21g; Fiber: 8g; Sugar: 1g; Protein: 30g; Sodium: 319mg; Cholesterol: 46mg

LEMON PESTO SALMON

Prep Time: 5 minutes / Cook Time: 10 minutes / Serves 2

30 minutes, gluten-free

I used to think of pesto as a topping for pasta, but then I discovered it's actually the most amazing, multipurpose condiment ever! I stir it into plain Greek yogurt to make a dip, add it to soups to zip up the flavor, and mix it with olive oil and vinegar for a pesto vinaigrette. It's also a perfect grilling sauce for chicken or fish. I often make this Lemon Pesto Salmon and serve it over a green salad with a drizzle of pesto vinaigrette.

10 ounces salmon fillet (1 large piece or 2 smaller ones)

Salt

Freshly ground black pepper

2 tablespoons prepared pesto sauce

1 large fresh lemon, sliced

1. Oil the grill grate and heat the grill to medium-high heat. Alternatively, you can roast the salmon in a 350°F oven.

2. Prepare the salmon by seasoning with salt and freshly ground black pepper, and then spread the pesto sauce on top.

3. Make a bed of fresh lemon slices about the same size as your fillet on the hot grill (or on a baking sheet if roasting), and rest the salmon on top of the lemon slices. Place any additional lemon slices on top of the salmon.

4. Grill the salmon for 6 to 10 minutes, or until it's opaque and flakes apart easily. If roasting, it will take about 20 minutes. There is no need to flip the fish over.

PREP TIP: Salmon should be cooked to an internal temperature of 145°F. Keep in mind that a thicker piece of fish will take longer to cook.

INGREDIENT TIP: When purchasing pesto, check the ingredients to make sure it's made with olive oil and not corn or soybean oil. Also check to see if it contains salt—if so, you'll need less salt to season your salmon.

Per Serving: Calories: 315; Total fat: 21g; Total carbs: 1g; Fiber: 0g; Sugar: 1g; Protein: 29g; Sodium: 176mg; Cholesterol: 84mg

SHRIMP WITH ARUGULA PESTO AND ZUCCHINI NOODLES

Prep Time: 20 minutes / Cook Time: 5 minutes / Serves 2

30 minutes, gluten-free

Pesto doesn't have to be made from basil alone, and zucchini can be transformed into pasta—who knew? You can make pesto from practically any herbs or greens you have on hand, or from sun-dried tomatoes or roasted red peppers. Here I used arugula, which makes a zesty topping for zucchini noodles in this low-carb and veggie-packed meal. Purchase cooked shrimp and zucchini noodles from the produce or freezer section of the grocery store for a quick, almost no-cook meal.

3 cups lightly packed arugula

½ cup lightly packed basil leaves

3 medium garlic cloves

¼ cup walnuts

3 tablespoons olive oil

2 tablespoons grated Parmesan cheese

1 tablespoon freshly squeezed lemon juice

Salt

Freshly ground black pepper

1 (10-ounce) package zucchini noodles

8 ounces cooked, shelled shrimp

2 Roma tomatoes, diced

1. Combine the arugula, basil, garlic, walnuts, olive oil, Parmesan cheese, and lemon juice in a food processor fitted with the chopping blade. Process until smooth, scraping down the sides as needed. Season with salt and pepper.

2. Heat a sauté pan over medium heat. Add the pesto, zucchini noodles, and shrimp. Toss to combine the sauce over the noodles and shrimp, and cook until warmed through. Don't overcook or the zucchini will become limp.

3. Taste and add additional salt and pepper if needed. Top with the diced tomatoes.

VARIATION TIP: To make this dairy-free, substitute nutritional yeast for the Parmesan cheese.

PREP TIP: If you don't have a food processor, use a blender to make the pesto. Just make sure you scrape down the sides often.

Per Serving: Calories: 434; Total fat: 30g; Total carbs: 15g; Fiber: 5g; Sugar: 7g; Protein: 33g; Sodium: 412mg; Cholesterol: 154mg

SALMON CAKES WITH TZATZIKI SAUCE

Prep Time: 10 minutes / Cook Time: 15 minutes, plus 20 minutes to cook the salmon if necessary / Serves 2

30 minutes

Salmon is my go-to fish, because it's so readily available and it's such a good source of those heart- and brain-healthy omega-3 fatty acids. I like to eat it at least once or twice each week. If I buy too much, salmon cakes are a perfect way to use up the extra cooked salmon. They freeze well for a night when you don't feel like cooking. Serve them over greens for a light dinner.

For the tzatziki sauce

½ cup plain Greek yogurt

1 teaspoon dried dill

¼ cup minced cucumber

Salt

Freshly ground black pepper

For the salmon cakes

6 ounces cooked salmon (or 8 ounces raw)

3 tablespoons olive oil, divided

¼ cup minced celery

¼ cup minced onion

½ teaspoon dried dill

1 tablespoon fresh minced parsley

Salt

Freshly ground black pepper

1 egg, beaten

½ cup unseasoned bread crumbs

To make the tzatziki sauce
Combine the yogurt, dill, and cucumber in a small bowl. Season with salt and pepper and set aside.

To make the salmon cakes

1. Remove any skin from the salmon. Place the salmon in a medium bowl and break it into small flakes with a fork. Set it aside.

2. Heat 1 tablespoon of olive oil in a nonstick skillet over medium-high heat. Add the celery and onion and sauté for 5 minutes.

3. Add the celery and onion to the salmon and stir to combine. Add the dill and parsley, and season with salt and pepper.

4. Add the beaten egg and bread crumbs and stir until mixed thoroughly.

5. Wipe the skillet clean and add the remaining 2 tablespoons of oil. Heat the pan over medium-high heat.

6. Form the salmon mixture into 4 patties, and place them two at a time into the hot pan.

7. Cook for 3 minutes per side, or until they're golden brown. Carefully flip them over with a spatula and cook for another 3 minutes on the second side.

8. Repeat with the remaining salmon cakes and serve topped with the tzatziki sauce.

PREP TIP: If you are starting with raw salmon, roast a salmon fillet in a 350°F oven for 20 minutes, or until fish flakes easily. Then, proceed with the rest of the recipe as written.

INGREDIENT TIP: If you prefer, you can make these with canned salmon instead of fresh.

Per Serving: Calories: 555; Total fat: 41g; Total carbs: 18g; Fiber: 2g; Sugar: 4g; Protein: 31g; Sodium: 303mg; Cholesterol: 146mg

PAN-ROASTED WILD COD WITH TOMATOES, OLIVES, AND ARTICHOKES

Prep Time: 10 minutes / Cook Time: 20 minutes / Serves 2

30 minutes, dairy-free, gluten-free

Even though cod is very lean and low in fat, it still adds some omega-3 fatty acids to your diet. The wonderful thing about this meal is that it comes together in minutes and cooks right on the stovetop in just a few more. It's also got a full serving of vegetables right in the pan. Add a side of Toasted Grain and Almond Pilaf (page 161) if you like.

1 tablespoon olive oil

½ medium onion, minced

2 garlic cloves, minced

1 teaspoon oregano

1 (15-ounce) can diced tomatoes with basil

1 (15-ounce) can artichoke hearts in water, drained and halved

¼ cup pitted Greek olives, drained

10 ounces wild cod (2 smaller pieces may fit better in the pan)

Salt

Freshly ground black pepper

1. Heat olive oil in a sauté pan over medium-high heat. Add the onion and sauté for about 10 minutes, or until golden. Add the garlic and oregano and cook for another 30 seconds.

2. Mix in the tomatoes, artichoke hearts, and olives.

3. Place the cod on top of the vegetables. Cover the pan and cook for 10 minutes, or until the fish is opaque and flakes apart easily. Season with salt and pepper.

SUBSTITUTION TIP: You can easily substitute any lean whitefish for the cod in this recipe.

Per Serving: Calories: 333; Total fat: 11g; Total carbs: 31g; Fiber: 8g; Sugar: 12g; Protein: 29g; Sodium: 1907mg; Cholesterol: 69mg

ROASTED BRANZINO WITH LEMON AND HERBS

Prep Time: 10 minutes / Cook Time: 20 minutes / Serves 2
30 minutes, dairy-free, gluten-free

Branzino (or branzini) is a small Mediterranean fish that's scaled and gutted by your fishmonger and usually cooked whole, with the tail and head intact. They're usually farmed, but are a good, sustainable option. Branzino may also be labeled as Mediterranean sea bass.

1 to 1½ pounds branzino, scaled and gutted

Salt

Freshly ground black pepper

1 tablespoon olive oil

1 lemon, sliced

3 garlic cloves, minced

¼ cup chopped fresh herbs (any mixture of oregano, thyme, parsley, and rosemary)

1. Preheat the oven to 425°F and set the rack to the middle position.

2. Lay the cleaned fish in a baking dish and make 4 to 5 slits in it, about 1½ inches apart.

3. Season the inside of the branzino with salt and pepper and drizzle with olive oil.

4. Fill the cavity of the fish with lemon slices. Sprinkle the chopped garlic and herbs over the lemon and close the fish.

5. Roast the fish for 15 to 20 minutes, or until the flesh is opaque and it flakes apart easily.

6. Before eating, open the fish, remove the lemon slices, and carefully pull out the bone.

INGREDIENT TIP: To ensure freshness, always buy fish from a reputable market and, ideally, cook it the day you buy it. Fresh fish should smell like the ocean, not overly fishy. A whole fish should have bright, bulging eyes and pink gills.

Per Serving: Calories: 287; Total fat: 12g; Total carbs: 2g; Fiber: 0g; Sugar: 0g; Protein: 42g; Sodium: 151mg; Cholesterol: 90mg

SUMMER MACKEREL NIÇOISE PLATTER

Prep Time: 10 minutes / Cook Time: 15 minutes / Serves 2

30 minutes, dairy-free, gluten-free

I have yet to visit the south of France, but when I get there, I guarantee you I'll have one of these salads! This is such a perfect light dinner for a warm night when you want something simple but satisfying. A Niçoise salad traditionally includes Niçoise olives, hard-boiled eggs, and an oily fish—typically tuna, but any fatty fish you have on hand works. I like to keep it simple by using canned mackerel fillets. Mackerel is a sustainable fish that's extremely high in omega-3 fatty acids.

For the dressing

3 tablespoons red wine vinegar

4 tablespoons olive oil

1 teaspoon Dijon mustard

¼ teaspoon salt

Pinch freshly ground black pepper

For the salad

2 teaspoons salt

2 small red potatoes

1 cup tender green beans

2 cups baby greens

2 hard-boiled eggs

½ cup cherry tomatoes, halved

⅓ cup Niçoise olives

2 (4-ounce) tins of mackerel fillets, drained

To make the dressing

Combine the vinegar, olive oil, Dijon mustard, salt, and pepper in a lidded jar. Shake or whisk the dressing until thoroughly combined. Taste and add more salt and pepper to taste, if needed.

To make the salad

1. Fill a large saucepan with about 3 inches of water, add salt, and bring to a boil. Add the potatoes and cook for 10 to 15 minutes, or until you can pierce them with a sharp knife, but they are still firm.

2. Remove the potatoes and add the green beans to the water. Reduce the heat and let the beans simmer for 5 minutes.

3. Place both the potatoes and green beans in a colander and run it under cold water until vegetables are cool.

4. Lay the baby greens on a large platter.

5. Slice the potatoes and arrange them on one section of the platter. Add the green beans to another section of the platter. Slice the hard-boiled eggs and arrange them in another section.

6. Continue with the tomatoes, olives, and mackerel fillets. Pour the dressing over the salad.

VARIATION TIP: This is a flexible, anything-goes kind of a salad, so if you have cucumbers, radishes, or even some grilled corn available, feel free to add or substitute any ingredients. You can also use canned tuna, grilled salmon, or even grilled chicken instead of the mackerel.

INGREDIENT TIP: I love the quality and taste of Wild Planet Foods canned mackerel.

Per Serving: Calories: 657; Total fat: 47g; Total carbs: 38g; Fiber: 7g; Sugar: 4g; Protein: 25g; Sodium: 355mg; Cholesterol: 164mg

SIMPLE POACHED SALMON WITH MUSTARD-HERB SAUCE

Prep Time: 15 minutes / Cook Time: 15 minutes / Serves 2

30 minutes, gluten-free

Poaching is the easiest and, I think, the most foolproof way to cook fish. Because the fish cooks slowly in some liquid, it's almost impossible to over-cook it or dry it out. I love the combination of salmon and mustard sauce, with a pop of flavor from some dried tarragon.

For the mustard-herb sauce

¼ cup plain Greek yogurt

2 tablespoons grainy Dijon mustard

1½ teaspoons dried tarragon

Pinch salt

Pinch freshly ground black pepper

For the salmon

10 ounces salmon fillet (1 large piece or 2 smaller ones)

1 tablespoon olive oil

Salt

Freshly ground black pepper

½ fresh lemon, sliced

Juice of ½ lemon

¼ cup dry white wine

¼ cup water

To make the mustard-herb sauce

Combine the yogurt, mustard, tarragon, salt, and pepper in a small bowl. Set aside.

To make the salmon

1. Rub the salmon with olive oil, and season with salt and pepper. Place the lemon slices on top.

2. In a sauté pan with a tight-fitting lid, bring the lemon juice, wine, and water to a boil. Gently slide the salmon into the pan.

3. Cover, reduce the heat to medium, and let the salmon simmer for 15 minutes, or until fish is opaque and flakes easily.

4. Remove salmon from the pan and divide between two plates. Top with the mustard sauce and serve.

SUBSTITUTION TIP: You can substitute oregano, thyme, or rosemary for the tarragon.

Per Serving: Calories: 332; Total fat: 21g; Total carbs: 3g; Fiber: 0g; Sugar: 2g; Protein: 23g; Sodium: 449mg; Cholesterol: 71mg

GRILLED HALIBUT STEAKS WITH ROMESCO SAUCE

Prep Time: 20 minutes / Cook Time: 10 minutes / Serves 2

30 minutes, dairy-free, gluten-free

Romesco is one of those multipurpose sauces that makes everything it touches taste better. It's also jam-packed with flavor, antioxidants from the bright peppers and sun-dried tomatoes, and healthy fats from almonds and olive oil.

For the romesco sauce

½ cup jarred roasted piquillo peppers

2 tablespoons sun-dried tomatoes in olive oil with herbs

2 small garlic cloves

¼ cup raw, unsalted almonds

2 tablespoons red wine vinegar

Pinch salt

¼ teaspoon smoked paprika (or more to taste)

¼ cup olive oil

1 to 2 tablespoons water

For the halibut

2 (5-ounce) halibut steaks

1 tablespoon olive oil

Salt

Freshly ground black pepper

To make the romesco sauce

1. Combine the piquillo peppers, sun-dried tomatoes, garlic, almonds, vinegar, salt, and paprika in a food processor or a blender and blend until mostly smooth. While the mixture is blending, drizzle in the olive oil.

2. Taste and adjust seasonings. If you prefer a smoother sauce, add water, 1 tablespoon at a time, until sauce reaches your desired consistency.

To make the salmon

1. Heat the grill to medium-high (350–400°F) and oil the grill grates.

2. Brush the fish with olive oil, and season with salt and pepper.

3. When the grill is hot, grill the fish for about 5 minutes per side, or until it's opaque and flakes easily. Serve topped with a few tablespoons of the romesco sauce.

4. Store any remaining sauce in an airtight container in the refrigerator for up to a week.

Per Serving: Calories: 264; Total fat: 13g; Total carbs: 3g; Fiber: 1g; Sugar: 1g; Protein: 31g; Sodium: 109mg; Cholesterol: 0mg

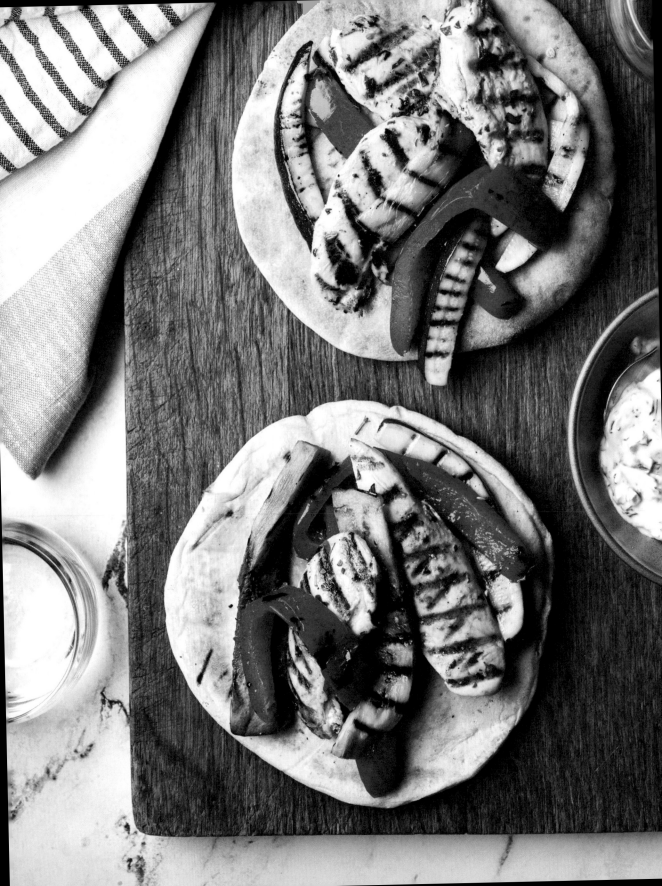

CHAPTER 8

POULTRY MAINS

Poultry is a part of the Mediterranean diet, but it's enjoyed less frequently than seafood or vegetarian meals. In addition, portion sizes are on the smaller side because they're accompanied by generous servings of vegetables and, often, beans or grains.

Much like fish or eggs, poultry is a great protein choice because it's quick cooking and quite high in protein, B vitamins, and iron. When buying poultry, look for packages labeled "pasture-raised." It can be more expensive, but this is a good time to go for quality over quantity. When preparing poultry, make sure you remove the skin before eating it—it's better for your heart.

< Chicken Gyros with Grilled Vegetables and Tzatziki Sauce, page 118

CHICKEN CUTLETS WITH GREEK SALSA

Prep Time: 15 minutes, plus 30 minutes to rest / Cook Time: 15 minutes / Serves 2
gluten-free

Everyone should have an herb garden, even if it's just a few small pots near your kitchen window. Herbs not only add flavor to your cooking, they're also full of disease-fighting antioxidants. This dish features simple ingredients that shine, and using herbs from your own garden makes it taste even better! I like to let the Greek salsa rest for about 30 minutes so the flavors can really develop. Be sure to taste the dish before seasoning with salt; the feta cheese and olives add a lot of saltiness to the dish.

2 tablespoons olive oil, divided

¼ teaspoon salt, plus additional to taste

Zest of ½ lemon

Juice of ½ lemon

8 ounces of chicken cutlets, or chicken breast sliced through the middle to make 2 thin pieces

1 cup cherry or grape tomatoes, halved or quartered (about 4 ounces)

½ cup minced red onion (about ⅓ medium onion)

1 medium cucumber, peeled, seeded and diced (about 1 cup)

5 to 10 pitted Greek olives, minced (more or less depending on size and your taste)

1. In a medium bowl, combine 1 tablespoon of olive oil, the salt, lemon zest, and lemon juice. Add the chicken and let it marinate while you make the salsa.

2. In a small bowl, combine the tomatoes, onion, cucumber, olives, parsley, oregano, mint, feta cheese, and red wine vinegar, and toss lightly. Cover and let rest in the refrigerator for at least 30 minutes. Taste the salsa before serving and add a pinch of salt or extra herbs if desired.

3. To cook the chicken, heat the remaining 1 tablespoon of olive oil in a large nonstick skillet over medium-high heat. Add the chicken pieces and cook for 3 to 6 minutes on each side, depending on the thickness. If the chicken sticks to the pan, it's not quite ready to flip.

4. When chicken is cooked through, top with the salsa and serve.

1 tablespoon minced
fresh parsley

1 tablespoon minced
fresh oregano

1 tablespoon minced
fresh mint

1 ounce crumbled
feta cheese

1 tablespoon red
wine vinegar

PREP TIP: The chicken can also be grilled instead
of pan-fried.

SUBSTITUTION TIP: Dried herbs can be substituted in the
salsa if you don't have fresh herbs on hand (although fresh
parsley really makes a difference). If you use dried herbs, use
only ½ tablespoon of each.

Per Serving: Calories: 357; Total fat: 23g; Total carbs: 8g;
Fiber: 2g; Sugar: 5g; Protein: 31g; Sodium: 202mg;
Cholesterol: 90mg

GREEK YOGURT–MARINATED CHICKEN BREASTS

Prep Time: 15 minutes, plus 30 minutes to marinate /
Cook Time: 30 minutes / Serves 2

gluten-free

I always have plain Greek yogurt on hand because it's a versatile ingredient that can be combined with either sweet or savory ingredients. It's packed with protein, so it's a great addition to breakfast or an energizing afternoon snack. Yogurt is also my secret ingredient in so many marinades for chicken. The lactic acid gently tenderizes the chicken and the natural sugars in yogurt add a lovely caramelization to the outside of the meat.

½ cup plain Greek yogurt

3 garlic cloves, minced

2 tablespoons minced fresh oregano (or 1 tablespoon dried oregano)

Zest of 1 lemon

1 tablespoon olive oil

½ teaspoon salt

2 (4-ounce) boneless, skinless chicken breasts

1. In a medium bowl, add the yogurt, garlic, oregano, lemon zest, olive oil, and salt and stir to combine. If the yogurt is very thick, you may need to add a few tablespoons of water or a squeeze of lemon juice to thin it a bit.

2. Add the chicken to the bowl and toss it in the marinade to coat it well. Cover and refrigerate the chicken for at least 30 minutes or up to overnight.

3. Preheat the oven to 350°F and set the rack to the middle position.

4. Place the chicken in a baking dish and roast for 30 minutes, or until chicken reaches an internal temperature of 165°F.

VARIATION TIP: Yogurt makes a great base for any marinade flavor. Just combine it with your favorite fresh or dried herbs or spices.

SUBSTITUTION TIP: If you don't have yogurt on hand, buttermilk works equally well.

Per Serving: Calories: 255; Total fat: 13g; Total carbs: 8g; Fiber: 2g; Sugar: 4g; Protein: 29g; Sodium: 694mg; Cholesterol: 78mg

BRUSCHETTA CHICKEN BURGERS

Prep Time: 15 minutes / Cook Time: 15 minutes / Serves 2

30 minutes, gluten-free

Tomato, basil, and mozzarella are such a perfect flavor combination. In this recipe, they're incorporated into ground chicken and grilled up like a burger. This recipe makes a healthy swap for a beef burger and is full of flavor. Serve these chicken burgers on ciabatta bread or on a bed of arugula with sliced fresh tomato and a drizzle of balsamic glaze (see the Strawberry Caprese Skewers, page 47).

1 tablespoon olive oil

3 tablespoons finely minced onion

2 garlic cloves, minced

1 teaspoon dried basil

¼ teaspoon salt

3 tablespoons minced sun-dried tomatoes packed in olive oil

8 ounces ground chicken breast

3 pieces small mozzarella balls (ciliegine), minced

1. Heat the grill to high heat (about 400°F) and oil the grill grates. Alternatively, you can cook these in a nonstick skillet.

2. Heat the olive oil in a small skillet over medium-high heat. Add the onion and garlic and sauté for 5 minutes, until softened. Stir in the basil. Remove from the heat and place in a medium bowl.

3. Add the salt, sun-dried tomatoes, and ground chicken and stir to combine. Mix in the mozzarella balls.

4. Divide the chicken mixture in half and form into two burgers, each about ¾-inch thick.

5. Place the burgers on the grill and cook for five minutes, or until golden on the bottom. Flip the burgers over and grill for another five minutes, or until they reach an internal temperature of 165°F.

CONTINUED >

6. If cooking the burgers in a skillet on the stovetop, heat a nonstick skillet over medium-high heat and add the burgers. Cook them for 5 to 6 minutes on the first side, or until golden brown on the bottom. Flip the burgers and cook for an additional 5 minutes, or until they reach an internal temperature of 165°F.

VARIATION TIP: If you're not in the mood for burgers, form the chicken mixture into small meatballs and eat them with tomato sauce and pasta. Panfry them or bake them in the oven at 350°F for 15 to 20 minutes.

Per Serving: Calories: 301; Total fat: 17g; Total carbs: 6g; Fiber: 1g; Sugar: 3g; Protein: 32g; Sodium: 725mg; Cholesterol: 92mg

STOVETOP CHICKEN CACCIATORE

Prep Time: 15 minutes / Cook Time: 2 hours / Serves 2
dairy-free

Skinless chicken thighs are perfect for this recipe because they'll retain more moisture than chicken breasts. They have great flavor and without the skin they're also low in saturated fat.

1½ pounds bone-in chicken thighs, skin removed

½ teaspoon salt, divided

2 tablespoons olive oil

½ large onion, thinly sliced

4 ounces baby bella mushrooms, sliced

1 red sweet pepper, cut into 1-inch pieces

1 fresh rosemary sprig

1 (15-ounce) can crushed fire-roasted tomatoes

½ cup dry red wine

1 teaspoon Italian herb seasoning

½ teaspoon garlic powder

3 tablespoons flour

1. Pat the chicken dry and season it with a generous pinch of salt.

2. Heat the olive oil in a Dutch oven over medium-high heat. Add the chicken and cook for 5 minutes on each side, or until it's lightly browned all over.

3. Add the onion, mushrooms, and sweet pepper to the pot and sauté for 5 minutes more. Add the rosemary, tomatoes, wine, Italian seasoning, garlic powder and remaining salt. Stir to combine.

4. Bring the mixture to a boil, then reduce the heat to low. Let simmer slowly for at least 1 hour, and up to 2 hours, stirring occasionally, until the chicken is tender and easily pulls away from the bone.

5. Measure out 1 cup of the sauce from the pot and place it into a bowl. Add the flour and whisk well to make a slurry. Make sure it doesn't have any lumps.

6. Increase the heat to medium-high and slowly whisk the slurry back into the pot. Stir until it comes to a boil and cook until the sauce thickens.

7. If desired, remove the chicken from the bones, shred it, and add it back to the sauce prior to serving.

Per Serving: Calories: 519; Total fat: 23g; Total carbs: 37g; Fiber: 6g; Sugar: 16g; Protein: 32g; Sodium: 485mg; Cholesterol: 120mg

CHICKEN GYROS WITH GRILLED VEGETABLES AND TZATZIKI SAUCE

**Prep Time: 15 minutes, plus 30 minutes to marinate /
Cook Time: 15 minutes / Serves 2**

This is an easy and flavorful recipe that really is quicker than it might seem, especially when you start with chicken tenders that have already been cut into strips and trimmed. If you can find the Greek style of pita bread that's puffy and flat, use it. Otherwise, use whole pitas, but roll them rather than cutting them in half and stuffing them.

For the chicken

2 tablespoons freshly squeezed lemon juice

2 tablespoons olive oil, divided, plus extra for oiling the grill

1 teaspoon minced fresh oregano, or ½ teaspoon dry oregano

½ teaspoon garlic powder

½ teaspoon salt, divided, plus more to season vegetables

8 ounces chicken tenders

1 small zucchini, cut into ½-inch strips lengthwise

1 small eggplant, cut into 1-inch strips lengthwise

½ red pepper, seeded and cut in half lengthwise

¾ cup plain Greek yogurt

½ English cucumber, peeled and minced

1 tablespoon minced fresh dill

2 (8-inch) pita breads

1. In a medium bowl, combine the lemon juice, 1 tablespoon of olive oil, the oregano, garlic powder, and ¼ teaspoon of salt. Add the chicken and marinate for 30 minutes.

2. Place the zucchini, eggplant, and red pepper in a large mixing bowl and sprinkle liberally with salt and the remaining 1 tablespoon of olive oil. Toss them well to coat. Let the vegetables rest while the chicken is marinating.

3. In a medium bowl, combine the yogurt, the cucumber, the remaining salt, and the dill. Stir well to combine and set aside in the refrigerator.

4. When ready to grill, heat the grill to medium-high (350–400°F) and oil the grill grate.

5. Drain any liquid from the vegetables and place them on the grill. Remove the chicken tenders from the marinade and place them on the grill.

6. Cook chicken and vegetables for 3 minutes per side, or until the chicken is no longer pink inside and the vegetables have grill marks.

7. Remove the chicken and vegetables from the grill and set aside. On the grill, heat the pitas for about 30 seconds, flipping them frequently so they don't burn.

8. Divide the chicken tenders and vegetables between the pitas and top each with ¼ cup of the tzatziki sauce. Roll the pitas up like a cone to eat.

VARIATION TIP: This is also great if you grill the chicken and vegetables ahead of time and enjoy it cold. You can also vary the vegetables: Try a portobello mushroom, sweet onion slices, or summer squash.

Per Serving: Calories: 587; Total fat: 22g; Total carbs: 62g; Fiber: 12g; Sugar: 18g; Protein: 39g; Sodium: 954mg; Cholesterol: 84mg

SKILLET GREEK TURKEY AND RICE

Prep Time: 20 minutes / Cook Time: 30 minutes / Serves 2
dairy-free, gluten-free

Ground turkey is a nice change from chicken, especially when it can be pre-pared as a simple one-pan meal. When buying ground turkey, check the label to make sure it's low in fat, or look for the words "turkey breast," on the label. Ground turkey *breast* should only have about 3 grams of fat per 4-ounce serving. Some packages labeled "ground turkey" may have upwards of 17 grams of fat per serving because they contain dark meat and skin.

1 tablespoon olive oil

½ medium onion, minced

2 garlic cloves, minced

8 ounces ground turkey breast

½ cup roasted red peppers, chopped (about 2 jarred peppers)

¼ cup sun-dried tomatoes, minced

1 teaspoon dried oregano

½ cup brown rice

1¼ cups low-sodium chicken stock

Salt

2 cups lightly packed baby spinach

1. Heat the olive oil in a sauté pan over medium heat. Add the onion and sauté for 5 minutes. Add the garlic and cook for another 30 seconds.

2. Add the turkey breast and cook for 7 minutes, breaking the turkey up with a spoon, until no longer pink.

3. Add the roasted red peppers, sun-dried tomatoes, and oregano and stir to combine. Add the rice and chicken stock and bring the mixture to a boil.

4. Cover the pan and reduce the heat to medium-low. Simmer for 30 minutes, or until the rice is cooked and tender. Season with salt.

5. Add the spinach to the pan and stir until it wilts slightly.

INGREDIENT TIP: My favorite jarred roasted red peppers are piquillo peppers. They're a bit smaller than some other types and have a nice smoky-sweet flavor.

Per Serving: Calories: 446; Total fat: 17g; Total carbs: 49g; Fiber: 5g; Sugar: 6g; Protein: 30g; Sodium: 663mg; Cholesterol: 80mg

LEMON AND PAPRIKA HERB-MARINATED CHICKEN

Prep Time: 10 minutes, plus 30 minutes to marinate / Cook Time: 15 minutes / Serves 2

dairy-free, gluten-free

I've always wanted a lemon tree in my backyard, so when I moved to a warm climate a few years ago it was one of the first things that went into the yard. This simple lemon and herb marinade is one of my favorite ways to use fresh lemons; it gives grilled chicken so much flavor and makes it amazingly tender.

2 tablespoons olive oil

4 tablespoons freshly squeezed lemon juice

¼ teaspoon salt

1 teaspoon paprika

1 teaspoon dried basil

½ teaspoon dried thyme

¼ teaspoon garlic powder

2 (4-ounce) boneless, skinless chicken breasts

1. In a bowl with a lid, combine the olive oil, lemon juice, salt, paprika, basil, thyme, and garlic powder.

2. Add the chicken and marinate for at least 30 minutes, or up to 4 hours.

3. When ready to cook, heat the grill to medium-high (about 350–400°F) and oil the grill grate. Alternately, you can also cook these in a nonstick sauté pan over medium-high heat.

4. Grill the chicken for 6 to 7 minutes, or until it lifts away from the grill easily. Flip it over and grill for another 6 to 7 minutes, or until it reaches an internal temperature of 165°F.

PREP TIP: When grilling (or panfrying) chicken breasts, don't disturb them for a few minutes. If they don't lift off the grill easily, they're not done yet!

Per Serving: Calories: 252; Total fat: 16g; Total carbs: 2g; Fiber: 1g; Sugar: 1g; Protein: 27g; Sodium: 372mg; Cholesterol: 65mg

SKILLET CREAMY TARRAGON CHICKEN AND MUSHROOMS

Prep Time: 10 minutes / **Cook Time:** 20 minutes / Serves 2

30 minutes

Cream sauces make even the simplest dishes taste more luxurious. I always keep some full-fat plain Greek yogurt on hand to stir into a sauce like this. It's rich and creamy, but it has the benefit of being a healthy, fermented dairy food.

2 tablespoons olive oil, divided

½ medium onion, minced

4 ounces baby bella (cremini) mushrooms, sliced

2 small garlic cloves, minced

8 ounces chicken cutlets

2 teaspoons tomato paste

2 teaspoons dried tarragon

2 cups low-sodium chicken stock

6 ounces pappardelle pasta

¼ cup plain full-fat Greek yogurt

Salt

Freshly ground black pepper

1. Heat 1 tablespoon of the olive oil in a sauté pan over medium-high heat. Add the onion and mushrooms and sauté for 5 minutes. Add the garlic and cook for 1 minute more.

2. Move the vegetables to the edges of the pan and add the remaining 1 tablespoon of olive oil to the center of the pan. Place the cutlets in the center and let them cook for about 3 minutes, or until they lift up easily and are golden brown on the bottom.

3. Flip the chicken and cook for another 3 minutes.

4. Mix in the tomato paste and tarragon. Add the chicken stock and stir well to combine everything. Bring the stock to a boil.

5. Add the pappardelle. Break up the pasta if needed to fit into the pan. Stir the noodles so they don't stick to the bottom of the pan.

6. Cover the sauté pan and reduce the heat to medium-low. Let the chicken and noodles simmer for 15 minutes, stirring occasionally, until the pasta is cooked and the liquid is mostly absorbed. If the liquid absorbs too quickly and the pasta isn't cooked, add more water or chicken stock, about ¼ cup at a time as needed.

7. Remove the pan from the heat.

8. Stir 2 tablespoons of the hot liquid from the pan into the yogurt. Pour the tempered yogurt into the pan and stir well to mix it into the sauce. Season with salt and pepper.

9. The sauce will tighten up as it cools, so if it seems too thick, add a few tablespoons of water.

PREP TIP: When adding yogurt to a hot sauce, it's always a good idea to temper it first by stirring some of the hot cooking liquid in with the dairy ingredient. This helps to prevent curdling.

Per Serving: Calories: 556; Total fat: 18g; Total carbs: 56g; Fiber: 2g; Sugar: 4g; Protein: 42g; Sodium: 190mg; Cholesterol: 130mg

SHEET PAN PESTO CHICKEN WITH CRISPY GARLIC POTATOES

Prep Time: 15 minutes / Cook Time: 50 minutes / Serves 2

gluten-free

If the thing you hate most about cooking is washing dishes, a sheet pan dinner is for you! The trick is in the timing. Proteins like chicken or fish take much less time than hard vegetables like potatoes or carrots. For this meal, I start the potatoes first, and at a much higher temperature, which gives them a nice crispiness. Then turn down the heat and add the chicken for the last 30 minutes.

12 ounces small red potatoes (3 or 4 potatoes)

1 tablespoon olive oil

¼ teaspoon salt

½ teaspoon garlic powder

1 (8-ounce) boneless, skinless chicken breast

3 tablespoons prepared pesto

1. Preheat the oven to 425°F and set the rack to the bottom position. Line a baking sheet with parchment paper. (Do not use foil, as the potatoes will stick.)

2. Scrub the potatoes and dry them well, then dice into 1-inch pieces.

3. In a medium bowl, combine the potatoes, olive oil, salt, and garlic powder. Toss well to coat.

4. Place the potatoes on the parchment paper and roast for 10 minutes. Flip the potatoes and return to the oven for another 10 minutes.

5. While the potatoes are roasting, place the chicken in the same bowl and toss with the pesto, coating the chicken evenly.

6. Check the potatoes to make sure they are golden brown on the top and bottom. Toss them again and add the chicken breast to the pan.

7. Turn the heat down to 350°F and let the chicken and potatoes roast for 30 minutes. Check to make sure the chicken reaches an internal temperature of 165°F and the potatoes are tender inside.

INGREDIENT TIP: I prefer to use garlic powder on the potatoes in this recipe because fresh garlic will burn during the 50 minutes the potatoes are roasting. If you want to use fresh minced garlic, omit the garlic powder and toss the minced garlic with the potatoes about 5 minutes before removing them from the oven.

Per Serving: Calories: 377; Total fat: 16g; Total carbs: 31g; Fiber: 4g; Sugar: 2g; Protein: 30g; Sodium: 426mg; Cholesterol: 76mg

FARRO WITH CHICKEN SAUSAGE AND SUN-DRIED TOMATOES

Prep Time: 10 minutes / Cook Time: 45 minutes / Serves 2

dairy-free

Farro is a native Mediterranean type of wheat grain that's packed with fiber and protein. I love the chewy texture and I find that toasting it a bit before cooking brings out even more of its nutty flavor. It's a great substitute for rice and makes a nice, hearty meal.

1 tablespoon olive oil

½ medium onion, diced

¼ cup julienned sun-dried tomatoes packed in olive oil and herbs

8 ounces hot Italian chicken sausage, removed from the casing

¾ cup farro

1½ cups low-sodium chicken stock

2 cups loosely packed arugula

4 to 5 large fresh basil leaves, sliced thin

Salt

1. Heat the olive oil in a sauté pan over medium-high heat. Add the onion and sauté for 5 minutes. Add the sun-dried tomatoes and chicken sausage, stirring to break up the sausage. Cook for 7 minutes, or until the sausage is no longer pink.

2. Stir in the farro. Let it toast for 3 minutes, stirring occasionally.

3. Add the chicken stock and bring the mixture to a boil. Cover the pan and reduce the heat to medium-low. Let it simmer for 30 minutes, or until the farro is tender.

4. Stir in the arugula and let it wilt slightly. Add the basil, and season with salt.

INGREDIENT TIP: Farro is almost always sold "semi-pearled," which means that some of the outer hull has been removed to make it quicker cooking. Be sure to check the label—if you buy whole farro, it will take about an hour to cook.

Per Serving: Calories: 491; Total fat: 19g; Total carbs: 53g; Fiber: 7g; Sugar: 4g; Protein: 31g; Sodium: 765mg; Cholesterol: 93mg

MEDITERRANEAN CHICKEN SALAD WRAPS

Prep Time: 15 minutes / Serves 2

30 minutes

Do you ever stop to pick up a rotisserie chicken and then realize you have no idea what to do with it? That's when these easy sandwiches come in to save the day. They take minutes to assemble but they're packed with so much delicious flavor. And there's no cooking required!

For the tzatziki sauce

½ cup plain Greek yogurt

1 tablespoon freshly squeezed lemon juice

1 teaspoon dried dill

Pinch garlic powder

Salt

Freshly ground black pepper

For the salad wraps

2 (8-inch) pita or naan bread

1 cup shredded chicken meat

2 cups mixed greens

2 roasted red bell peppers, sliced thin

½ English cucumber, peeled if desired and sliced thin

¼ cup pitted black olives

1 scallion, chopped

To make the tzatziki sauce

Combine the Greek yogurt, lemon juice, dill, and garlic powder in a small bowl and season with salt and pepper.

To make the wraps

1. On each piece of pita or naan bread, spread ¼ cup of the tzatziki sauce and arrange half the chicken, mixed greens, red pepper slices, cucumber, olives, and scallion.

2. Roll up the sandwiches and, if desired, wrap the bottom half of each sandwich in foil so it's easier to eat.

INGREDIENT TIP: Use any leftover rotisserie chicken to add to Avgolemono (Lemon Chicken Soup) (page 56), or Creamy Tomato Hummus Soup (page 53).

Per Serving: Calories: 429; Total fat: 11g; Total carbs: 51g; Fiber: 6g; Sugar: 10g; Protein: 31g; Sodium: 676mg; Cholesterol: 75mg

MOROCCAN-SPICED CHICKEN THIGHS WITH SAFFRON BASMATI RICE

Prep Time: 15 minutes / Cook Time: 15 minutes / Serves 2

30 minutes, dairy-free, gluten-free

Moroccan dishes have such a perfect blend of flavors and aromas from an array of spices that most Americans would never think to put together—but they sure do work. In addition to delighting your taste buds, these spices are also packed with antioxidants that protect your cells from oxidative damage. Make a big batch of this spice mix and you'll have it to use on chicken, fish, vegetables, or anything else.

For the chicken

½ teaspoon paprika

½ teaspoon cumin

½ teaspoon cinnamon

¼ teaspoon salt

¼ teaspoon garlic powder

¼ teaspoon ginger powder

¼ teaspoon coriander

⅛ teaspoon cayenne pepper (a pinch—or more if you like it spicy)

10 ounces boneless, skinless chicken thighs (about 4 pieces)

For the rice

1 tablespoon olive oil

½ small onion, minced

½ cup basmati rice

2 pinches saffron

¼ teaspoon salt

1 cup low-sodium chicken stock

To make the chicken

1. Preheat the oven to 350°F and set the rack to the middle position.

2. In a small bowl, combine the paprika, cumin, cinnamon, salt, garlic powder, ginger powder, coriander, and cayenne pepper. Add chicken thighs and toss, rubbing the spice mix into the chicken.

3. Place the chicken in a baking dish and roast it for 35 to 40 minutes, or until the chicken reaches an internal temperature of 165°F. Let the chicken rest for 5 minutes before serving.

To make the rice

1. While the chicken is roasting, heat the oil in a sauté pan over medium-high heat. Add the onion and sauté for 5 minutes.

2. Add the rice, saffron, salt, and chicken stock. Cover the pot with a tight-fitting lid and reduce the heat to low. Let the rice simmer for 15 minutes, or until it is light and fluffy and the liquid has been absorbed.

SUBSTITUTION: If you prefer boneless or bone-in chicken breasts, you can swap them for the thighs.

Per Serving: Calories: 401; Total fat: 10g; Total carbs: 41g; Fiber: 2g; Sugar: 1g; Protein: 37g; Sodium: 715mg; Cholesterol: 81mg

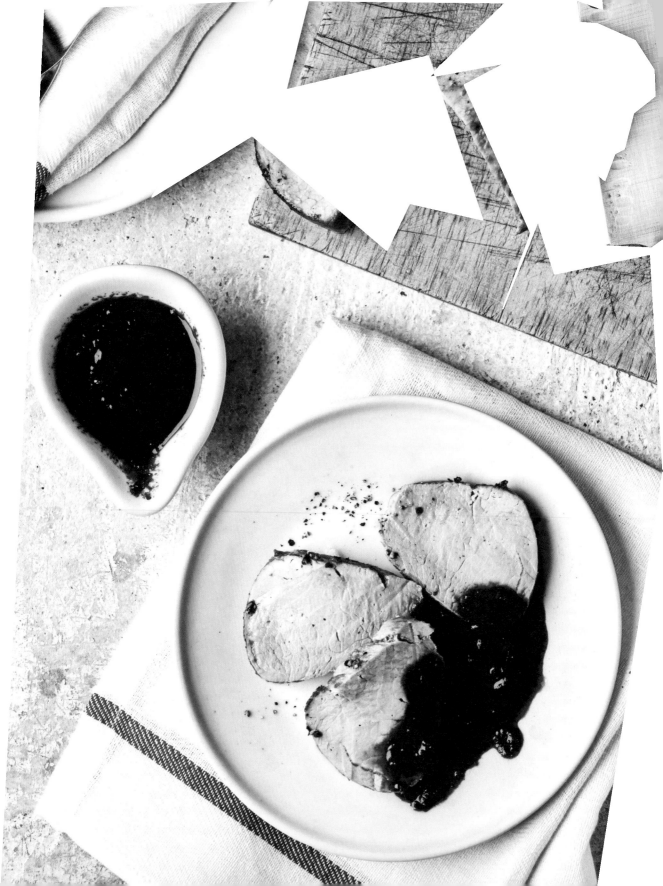

CHAPTER 9

BEEF, PORK, AND LAMB MAINS

Unlike the standard American diet, there is much less emphasis on meats like beef, pork, and lamb in the Mediterranean diet. It's not off limits, but it is usually reserved for special occasions. Because it takes more planning and time to prepare, and it's more expensive, I'm all in favor of meat moderation.

When it comes to meat, I always recommend going for quality over quantity. Whenever possible, purchase leaner cuts and grass-fed meats. They're more expensive, but better for you. Rather than choosing packaged meats that tend to come in larger quantities, choose smaller portions from the butcher counter—or divide a large package of meat into smaller portions before it goes into the freezer.

Instead of making a large serving of meat the star of your plate, treat meat like a condiment that adds flavor and complements the vegetables, whole grains, or legumes in your meal.

< Roast Pork Tenderloin with Cherry-Balsamic Sauce, page 143

SPICY LAMB BURGERS WITH HARISSA MAYO

Prep Time: 15 minutes / Cook Time: 10 minutes / Serves 2

30 minutes, dairy-free, gluten-free (without the bun)

Lamb is a part of the Mediterranean diet, although like beef it's eaten in moderation. Lamb has a different flavor than beef, but American-raised lamb is more tender and milder, less gamy than many people think. The flavor of lamb comes from its fat, so leaner cuts of lamb are milder tasting than those that are high in fat.

½ small onion, minced

1 garlic clove, minced

2 teaspoons minced fresh parsley

2 teaspoons minced fresh mint

¼ teaspoon salt

Pinch freshly ground black pepper

1 teaspoon cumin

1 teaspoon smoked paprika

¼ teaspoon coriander

8 ounces lean ground lamb

2 tablespoons olive oil mayonnaise

½ teaspoon harissa paste (more or less to taste)

2 hamburger buns or pitas, fresh greens, tomato slices (optional, for serving)

1. Preheat the grill to medium-high (350–400°F) and oil the grill grate. Alternatively, you can cook these in a heavy pan (cast iron is best) on the stovetop.

2. In a large bowl, combine the onion, garlic, parsley, mint, salt, pepper, cumin, paprika, and coriander. Add the lamb and, using your hands, combine the meat with the spices so they are evenly distributed. Form meat mixture into 2 patties.

3. Grill the burgers for 4 minutes per side, or until the internal temperature registers 160°F for medium.

4. If cooking on the stovetop, heat the pan to medium-high and oil the pan. Cook the burgers for 5 to 6 minutes per side, or until the internal temperature registers 160°F.

5. While the burgers are cooking, combine the mayonnaise and harissa in a small bowl.

6. Serve the burgers with the harissa mayonnaise and slices of tomato and fresh greens on a bun or pita—or skip the bun altogether.

SUBSTITUTION TIP: If you don't have harissa available, season your mayonnaise with ½ teaspoon of cumin and ½ teaspoon smoked paprika.

Per Serving: Calories: 381; Total fat: 20g; Total carbs: 27g; Fiber: 2g; Sugar: 4g; Protein: 22g; Sodium: 653mg; Cholesterol: 68mg

SLOW COOKER MEDITERRANEAN BEEF STEW

Prep Time: 20 minutes / Cook Time: 8 hours (slow cooker) or 3 hours (stovetop) / Serves 2, with leftovers for lunch

dairy-free

When the weather gets chilly, there's nothing like a pot of beef stew to warm you up. It smells wonderful as it's cooking all day, and it tastes even better. This is a Mediterranean version with a tomato, briny olive, and red wine sauce, using white beans and vegetables instead of the traditional carrots and potatoes. Because I think beef stew tastes even better the next day, this makes a bit more than two portions, so you can have leftovers for lunch tomorrow.

1 (15-ounce) can diced or crushed tomatoes with basil

1 teaspoon beef base or 1 beef bouillon cube

2 tablespoons olive oil, divided

8 ounces baby bella (cremini) mushrooms, quartered

½ large onion, diced

2 garlic cloves, minced

1 pound cubed beef stew meat

3 tablespoons flour

¼ teaspoon salt

Pinch freshly ground black pepper

¾ cup dry red wine

¼ cup minced brined olives

1 fresh rosemary sprig

1 (15-ounce) can white cannellini beans, drained and rinsed

1 medium zucchini, cut in half lengthwise and then cut into 1-inch pieces.

1. Pour the can of tomatoes into a slow cooker and set it to low heat. Add the beef base and stir to combine.

2. Heat 1 tablespoon of olive oil in a large sauté pan over medium heat. Add the mushrooms and onion and sauté for 10 minutes, or until they're golden. Add the garlic and cook for another 30 seconds. Transfer the vegetables to the slow cooker.

3. In a plastic food storage bag, combine the stew meat with the flour, salt, and pepper. Seal the bag and shake well to combine.

4. Heat the remining 1 tablespoon of oil in the sauté pan over high heat. Add the floured meat and sear to get a crust on the outside edges. Deglaze the pan by adding about half of the red wine and scraping up any browned bits on the bottom. Stir so the wine thickens a bit and transfer to the slow cooker along with any remaining wine.

5. Stir the stew to combine the ingredients. Add the olives and rosemary, cover, and cook for 6 to 8 hours on low.

6. About 30 minutes before the stew is finished, add the beans and zucchini to let them warm through.

PREP TIP: If you don't have a slow cooker, combine all of the ingredients in a Dutch oven and cook the stew on the stovetop over low heat, at a very slow simmer, for 2½ to 3 hours, or until the meat is fork-tender.

Per Serving: Calories: 388; Total fat: 15g; Total carbs: 25g; Fiber: 8g; Sugar: 6g; Protein: 31g; Sodium: 583mg; Cholesterol: 51mg

GREEK-STYLE GROUND BEEF PITA SANDWICHES

Prep Time: 15 minutes / Cook Time: 10 minutes / Serves 2

30 minutes

This meal is perfect for when you want something that's sandwich-quick, but a bit warmer and heartier. When buying ground beef, look for at least 90 percent lean, and, ideally, choose grass-fed beef. It has a healthier fat and nutrition profile compared to conventional beef.

For the beef

1 tablespoon olive oil

½ medium onion, minced

2 garlic cloves, minced

6 ounces lean ground beef

1 teaspoon dried oregano

For the yogurt sauce

⅓ cup plain Greek yogurt

1 ounce crumbled feta cheese (about 3 tablespoons)

1 tablespoon minced fresh parsley

1 tablespoon minced scallion

1 tablespoon freshly squeezed lemon juice

Pinch salt

For the sandwiches

2 large Greek-style pitas

½ cup cherry tomatoes, halved

1 cup diced cucumber

Salt

Freshly ground black pepper

To make the beef

Heat the olive oil in a sauté pan over medium high-heat. Add the onion, garlic, and ground beef and sauté for 7 minutes, breaking up the meat well. When the meat is no longer pink, drain off any fat and stir in the oregano. Turn off the heat.

To make the yogurt sauce

In a small bowl, combine the yogurt, feta, parsley, scallion, lemon juice, and salt.

To assemble the sandwiches

1. Warm the pitas in the microwave for 20 seconds each.

2. To serve, spread some of the yogurt sauce over each warm pita. Top with the ground beef, cherry tomatoes, and diced cucumber. Season with salt and pepper. Add additional yogurt sauce if desired.

SUBSTITUTION: If you prefer, you can make these with ground chicken or turkey breast instead of beef.

Per Serving: Calories: 541; Total fat: 21g; Total carbs: 57g; Fiber: 4g; Sugar: 9g; Protein: 29g; Sodium: 694mg; Cholesterol: 73mg

LEMON HERB-CRUSTED PORK TENDERLOIN

Prep Time: 10 minutes / Cook Time: 20 minutes / Serves 2

30 minutes, dairy-free, gluten-free

Pork tenderloin is an extremely lean, tender cut of meat that cooks in minutes, so it's perfect for a quick and easy dinner. I especially love the size. They're usually sold in 1 to 1½-pound packages with two smaller tenderloins in the package. Open it up when you bring it home and either freeze the second piece for a later date or make two different pork recipes for the week. It's a versatile meat that adapts to a variety of seasonings and sauces.

1 (8-ounce) pork tenderloin

Zest of 1 lemon

½ teaspoon dried thyme

¼ teaspoon garlic powder

¼ teaspoon za'atar seasoning

¼ teaspoon salt

1 tablespoon olive oil

1. Preheat the oven to 425°F and set the rack to the middle position.

2. Trim away any of the silver skin from the pork tenderloin, to prevent it from curling while it cooks.

3. Combine the lemon zest, thyme, garlic powder, za'atar, and salt in a small bowl. Rub it evenly over the pork tenderloin.

4. Heat the olive oil in a sauté pan over medium-high heat. Add the pork and sauté for 3 minutes, turning often, until it's golden on all sides.

5. Place the tenderloin in an oven-safe baking dish and roast for 15 minutes, or until the internal temperature registers 145°F. Remove it from the oven and let it rest for 3 minutes before serving.

PREP TIP: It's okay for pork tenderloin to be pink inside, as long as it's cooked to at least 145°F. Pork tenderloin is best served between 145° and 160°F. Because it's very lean, it can be too dry if cooked to a higher temperature.

Per Serving: Calories: 182; Total fat: 11g; Total carbs: 1g; Fiber: 0g; Sugar: 0g; Protein: 20g; Sodium: 356mg; Cholesterol: 65mg

ONE-PAN CREAMY ITALIAN SAUSAGE ORECCHIETTE

Prep Time: 5 minutes / Cook Time: 25 minutes / Serves 2
30 minutes

Orecchiette means "little ears" in Italian—referring to the shape of the pasta. I use orecchiette in this recipe because it soaks up the flavorful cream sauce. Italian sausage can be made from beef, pork, turkey, or chicken, or a combination of meats. There can also be a difference in the fat content, so check the label and buy one that's lower in saturated fat and minimally processed.

1 tablespoon olive oil

½ medium onion, diced

2 garlic cloves, minced

2 ounces baby bella (cremini) mushrooms, sliced

4 ounces hot or sweet Italian sausage

½ teaspoon Italian herb seasoning

1½ cups dry orecchiette pasta (about 6 ounces)

2 cups low-sodium chicken stock

2 cups packed baby spinach

¼ cup heavy cream

Salt

1. Heat the olive oil in a sauté pan over medium-high heat. Add the onion, garlic, and mushrooms and sauté for 5 minutes.

2. Remove the sausage from its casing and add it to the pan, breaking it up well. Cook for another 5 minutes, or until the sausage is no longer pink.

3. Add the Italian herb seasoning, pasta, and chicken stock. Bring the mixture to a boil.

4. Cover the pan, reduce the heat to medium-low, and let it simmer for 10 to 15 minutes, or until the pasta is cooked. Remove from the heat.

5. Add the spinach and stir it in to let it wilt.

6. Add the cream and season with salt. The sauce will tighten up as it cools. If it seems too thick, add additional chicken stock or water.

SUBSTITUTION TIP: You can substitute a small shell pasta for the orecchiette, and Italian turkey or chicken sausage for the regular Italian sausage.

Per Serving: Calories: 531; Total fat: 19g; Total carbs: 69g; Fiber: 5g; Sugar: 5g; Protein: 23g; Sodium: 569mg; Cholesterol: 38mg

PORK TENDERLOIN WITH CHERMOULA SAUCE

Prep Time: 15 minutes / Cook Time: 20 minutes / Serves 2
dairy-free, gluten-free

Chermoula is a North African or Moroccan herb and spice sauce that's delicious with so many different types of meat, fish, or even vegetables. There are many variations, but fresh parsley, cilantro, lemon, and garlic are fairly standard, along with some paprika and cumin.

½ cup fresh parsley

½ cup fresh cilantro

6 small garlic cloves

3 tablespoons olive oil, divided

3 tablespoons freshly squeezed lemon juice

1 teaspoon smoked paprika

2 teaspoons cumin

½ teaspoon salt, divided

Pinch freshly ground black pepper

1 (8-ounce) pork tenderloin

1. Preheat the oven to 425°F and set the rack to the middle position.

2. In the bowl of a food processor, combine the parsley, cilantro, garlic, 2 tablespoons of olive oil, the lemon juice, paprika, cumin, and ¼ teaspoon of salt. Pulse 15 to 20 times, or until the mixture is fairly smooth. Scrape the sides down as needed to incorporate all of the ingredients. Transfer the sauce to a small bowl and set aside.

3. Season the pork tenderloin on all sides with the remaining ¼ teaspoon of salt and a generous pinch of pepper.

4. Heat the remaining 1 tablespoon of olive oil in a sauté pan. Add the pork and sear for 3 minutes, turning often, until it's golden on all sides.

5. Transfer the pork to an oven-safe baking dish and roast for 15 minutes, or until the internal temperature registers 145°F.

VARIATION TIP: Other variations of chermoula sauce include ginger, cayenne pepper, saffron, turmeric, or sumac. Experiment with the flavors you like best.

Per Serving: Calories: 168; Total fat: 13g; Total carbs: 3g; Fiber: 1g; Sugar: 0g; Protein: 11g; Sodium: 333mg; Cholesterol: 33mg

GRILLED FILET MIGNON WITH RED WINE–MUSHROOM SAUCE

Prep Time: 20 minutes, plus 30 minutes for meat to come to room temperature / Cook Time: 20 minutes, plus 5 minutes to rest / Serves 2

dairy-free

There is no finer cut of meat (in my opinion) than filet mignon. It's an extremely lean cut of beef, but also incredibly tender. Because it's so low in fat, it doesn't have quite as much flavor as some other cuts. Once it's seasoned properly, however, it's amazing. I love herbes de Provence, a multipurpose herb seasoning that includes a variety of herbs native to the Provence region of southern France.

2 (3-ounce) pieces filet mignon

2 tablespoons olive oil, divided

8 ounces baby bella (cremini) mushrooms, quartered

1 large shallot, minced (about ⅓ cup)

2 teaspoons flour

2 teaspoons tomato paste

½ cup red wine

1 cup low-sodium chicken stock

½ teaspoon dried thyme

1 sprig fresh rosemary

1 teaspoon herbes de Provence

¼ teaspoon salt

¼ teaspoon garlic powder

¼ teaspoon onion powder

Pinch freshly ground black pepper

1. Preheat the oven to 425°F and set the oven rack to the middle position.

2. Remove the filets from the refrigerator about 30 minutes before you're ready to cook them. Pat them dry with a paper towel and let them rest while you prepare the mushroom sauce.

3. In a sauté pan, heat 1 tablespoon of olive oil over medium-high heat. Add the mushrooms and shallot and sauté for 10 minutes.

4. Add the flour and tomato paste and cook for another 30 seconds. Add the wine and scrape up any browned bits from the sauté pan. Add the chicken stock, thyme, and rosemary.

5. Stir the sauce so the flour doesn't form lumps and bring it to a boil. Once the sauce thickens, reduce the heat to the lowest setting and cover the pan to keep the sauce warm.

6. In a small bowl, combine the herbes de Provence, salt, garlic powder, onion powder, and pepper.

7. Rub the beef with the remaining 1 tablespoon of olive oil and season it on both sides with the herb mixture.

8. Heat an oven-safe sauté pan over medium-high heat. Add the beef and sear for 2½ minutes on each side. Then, transfer the pan to the oven for 5 more minutes to finish cooking. Use a meat thermometer to check the internal temperature and remove it at 130°F for medium-rare.

9. Tent the meat with foil and let it rest for 5 minutes before serving topped with the mushroom sauce.

PREP TIP: The cooking time on the meat will depend on the thickness. Make sure you keep a close eye on it and use a meat thermometer, to ensure it's cooked to your preferred temperature. The temperature will increase by a few degrees while the meat rests. The final temperature for medium-rare is 135°F; the final temperature for medium is 145°F.

INGREDIENT TIP: Herbes de Provence is available in the spice section of most grocery stores. It's an herb mix that includes savory, marjoram, rosemary, thyme, oregano, and lavender.

Per Serving: Calories: 385; Total fat: 20g; Total carbs: 15g; Fiber: 0g; Sugar: 5g; Protein: 25g; Sodium: 330mg; Cholesterol: 59mg

BAKED LAMB KOFTA MEATBALLS

Prep Time: 15 minutes / Cook Time: 30 minutes / Serves 2

dairy-free, gluten-free

Kofta might just be the most flavorful dish I've ever tasted, and it's so easy to make. It's often served on skewers, but I think it's easier to do as meatballs. Serve these meatballs on top of grains, pasta, greens, or in a pita with tzatziki sauce (see Chicken Gyros with Grilled Vegetables and Tzatziki Sauce, page 118). Whatever you choose, your taste buds won't be disappointed!

¼ cup walnuts

½ small onion

1 garlic clove

1 roasted piquillo pepper

2 tablespoons fresh parsley

2 tablespoons fresh mint

¼ teaspoon salt

¼ teaspoon cumin

¼ teaspoon allspice

Pinch cayenne pepper

8 ounces lean ground lamb

1. Preheat the oven to 350°F and set the rack to the middle position. Line a baking sheet with foil.

2. In the bowl of a food processor, combine the walnuts, onion, garlic, roasted pepper, parsley, mint, salt, cumin, allspice, and cayenne pepper. Pulse about 10 times to combine everything.

3. Transfer the spice mixture to the bowl and add the lamb. With your hands or a spatula, mix the spices into the lamb.

4. Roll into 1½-inch balls (about the size of golf balls).

5. Place the meatballs on the foil-lined baking sheet and bake for 30 minutes, or until cooked to an internal temperature of 160°F.

SUBSTITUTION TIP: If you don't have ground lamb on hand, lean ground beef is a good substitute.

Per Serving: Calories: 408; Total fat: 23g; Total carbs: 7g; Fiber: 3g; Sugar: 1g; Protein: 22g; Sodium: 429mg; Cholesterol: 80mg

ROAST PORK TENDERLOIN WITH CHERRY-BALSAMIC SAUCE

Prep Time: 20 minutes / Cook Time: 20 minutes, plus 5 minutes to rest / Serves 2

dairy-free, gluten-free

Frozen cherries are one of the fruits that I always have stocked in my freezer. They're a great source of vitamin C and potassium, and they're rich in antioxidants and compounds that reduce inflammation. They also happen to pair nicely with pork, especially in this sweet and tangy sauce.

1 cup frozen cherries, thawed

⅓ cup balsamic vinegar

1 fresh rosemary sprig

1 (8-ounce) pork tenderloin

¼ teaspoon salt

⅛ teaspoon freshly ground black pepper

1 tablespoon olive oil

1. Combine the cherries and vinegar in a blender and purée until smooth.

2. Pour into a saucepan, add the rosemary sprig, and bring the mixture to a boil. Reduce the heat to medium-low and simmer for 15 minutes, or until it's reduced by half.

3. While the sauce is simmering, preheat the oven to 425°F and set the rack in the middle position.

4. Season the pork on all sides with the salt and pepper.

5. Heat the oil in a sauté pan over medium-high heat. Add the pork and sear for 3 minutes, turning often, until it's golden on all sides.

6. Transfer the pork to an oven-safe baking dish and roast for 15 minutes, or until the internal temperature is 145°F.

7. Let the pork rest for 5 minutes before serving. Serve sliced and topped with the cherry-balsamic sauce.

Per Serving: Calories: 328; Total fat: 11g; Total carbs: 30g; Fiber: 1g; Sugar: 26g; Protein: 21g; Sodium: 386mg; Cholesterol: 65mg

GREEK-INSPIRED BEEF KEBABS

Prep Time: 15 minutes, plus 4 hours to marinate / Cook Time: 15 minutes / Serves 2
dairy-free, gluten-free

Beef and vegetable kebabs are full of color and flavor and make a perfect summer dinner to cook on the grill. Use whatever vegetables are available at the farmers' market and serve the kebabs with Toasted Grain and Almond Pilaf (page 161). While you can alternate the meat and vegetables on each skewer, I like to separate them, since the cooking time might vary.

6 ounces beef sirloin tip, trimmed of fat and cut into 2-inch pieces

3 cups of any mixture of vegetables: mushrooms, zucchini, summer squash, onions, cherry tomatoes, red peppers

½ cup olive oil

¼ cup freshly squeezed lemon juice

2 tablespoons balsamic vinegar

2 teaspoons dried oregano

1 teaspoon garlic powder

1 teaspoon minced fresh rosemary

1 teaspoon salt

1. Place the meat in a large shallow container or in a plastic freezer bag.

2. Cut the vegetables into similar-size pieces and place them in a second shallow container or freezer bag.

3. For the marinade, combine the olive oil, lemon juice, balsamic vinegar, oregano, garlic powder, rosemary, and salt in a measuring cup. Whisk well to combine. Pour half of the marinade over the meat, and the other half over the vegetables.

4. Place the meat and vegetables in the refrigerator to marinate for 4 hours.

5. When you are ready to cook, preheat the grill to medium-high (350–400°F) and grease the grill grate.

6. Thread the meat onto skewers and the vegetables onto separate skewers.

7. Grill the meat for 3 minutes on each side. They should only take 10 to 12 minutes to cook, but it will depend on how thick the meat is.

8. Grill the vegetables for about 3 minutes on each side or until they have grill marks and are softened.

INGREDIENT TIP: Sirloin tip needs a few hours of marinating time to tenderize it, but I think it's very flavorful for kebabs, and it's always reasonably priced.

PREP TIP: If you're using wooden skewers, soak them in a pan of water for 30 minutes while you're marinating the meat.

Per Serving: Calories: 285; Total fat: 18g; Total carbs: 9g; Fiber: 4g; Sugar: 4g; Protein: 21g; Sodium: 123mg; Cholesterol: 77mg

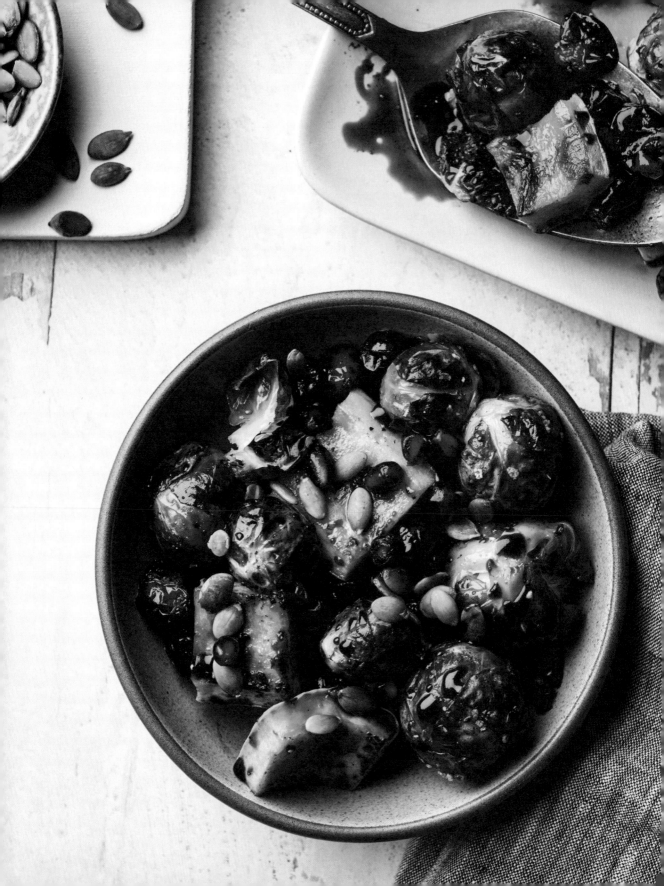

CHAPTER 10

SIMPLE SIDES

Side dishes can really make your meal shine by adding lots of colors, textures, and flavors. They complement the protein portion of your meal, and when they're full of the best parts of the Mediterranean diet—vegetables, whole grains, and legumes—they also enhance the nutrition content of your plate.

As a dietitian, one simple piece of advice I give to help people eat better is to eat a vegetable, any vegetable, every time you eat. It's something most of us struggle with, so I've included lots of easy vegetable options here to help you learn to love them. Roasting is my favorite way to prepare vegetables because it brings out a delicious sweetness that makes you appreciate them in a whole new way.

< Roasted Brussels Sprouts with Delicata Squash and Balsamic Glaze, page 154

LEMON-THYME ROASTED MIXED VEGETABLES

Prep Time: 20 minutes / Cook Time: 50 minutes / Serves 2

dairy-free, gluten-free, vegan, vegetarian

Too many people tell me they don't like vegetables. When I ask how they prepare them, and they tell me they use frozen vegetables and steam them, I understand why! Nothing against frozen vegetables and steaming, but once you use fresh vegetables and roast them with simple seasoning like garlic, lemon, and a few fresh herbs, you'll see what you're missing. This recipe makes two generous portions—which is a good thing.

1 head garlic, cloves split apart, unpeeled

2 tablespoons olive oil, divided

2 medium carrots

¼ pound asparagus

6 Brussels sprouts

2 cups cauliflower florets

½ pint cherry or grape tomatoes

½ fresh lemon, sliced

Salt

Freshly ground black pepper

3 sprigs fresh thyme or ½ teaspoon dried thyme

Freshly squeezed lemon juice

1. Preheat oven to 375°F and set the rack to the middle position. Line a sheet pan with parchment paper or foil.

2. Place the garlic cloves in a small piece of foil and wrap lightly to enclose them, but don't seal the package. Drizzle with 1 teaspoon of olive oil. Place the foil packet on the sheet pan and roast for 30 minutes while you prepare the remaining vegetables.

3. While garlic is roasting, clean, peel, and trim vegetables: Cut carrots into strips, ½-inch wide and 3 to 4 inches long; snap tough ends off asparagus; trim tough ends off the Brussels sprouts and cut in half if they are large; trim cauliflower into 2-inch florets; keep tomatoes whole. The vegetables should be cut into pieces of similar size for even roasting.

4. Place all vegetables and the lemon slices into a large mixing bowl. Drizzle with the remaining 5 teaspoons of olive oil and season generously with salt and pepper.

5. Increase the oven temperature to 400°F.

6. Arrange the vegetables on the sheet pan in a single layer, leaving the packet of garlic cloves on the pan. Roast for 20 minutes, turning occasionally, until tender.

7. When the vegetables are tender, remove from the oven and sprinkle with thyme leaves. Let the garlic cloves sit until cool enough to handle, and then remove the skins. Leave them whole, or gently mash.

8. Toss garlic with the vegetables and an additional squeeze of fresh lemon juice.

SUBSTITUTION TIP: You can use any vegetables you like in this recipe, as long as you cut them into pieces of about the same size.

Per Serving: Calories: 256; Total fat: 15g; Total carbs: 31g; Fiber: 9g; Sugar: 12g; Protein: 7g; Sodium: 168mg; Cholesterol: 0mg

CRISPY ROASTED RED POTATOES WITH GARLIC, ROSEMARY, AND PARMESAN

Prep Time: 10 minutes / Cook Time: 55 minutes / Serves 2
gluten-free, vegetarian

Many people avoid potatoes because of the carbs, but they're actually a great source of potassium, vitamin C, and fiber. The key is to keep your portion size on the small side. These do take some time to roast, but if you're patient they'll be perfectly crispy outside and soft inside. White potatoes do have a bigger impact on your blood sugar than sweet potatoes or purple potatoes, so feel free to substitute them.

12 ounces red potatoes (3 to 4 small potatoes)

1 tablespoon olive oil

½ teaspoon garlic powder

¼ teaspoon salt

1 tablespoon grated Parmesan cheese

1 teaspoon minced fresh rosemary (from 1 sprig)

1. Preheat the oven to 425°F and set the rack to the bottom position. Line a baking sheet with parchment paper. (Do not use foil, as the potatoes will stick.)

2. Scrub the potatoes and dry them well. Dice into 1-inch pieces.

3. In a mixing bowl, combine the potatoes, olive oil, garlic powder, and salt. Toss well to coat.

4. Lay the potatoes on the parchment paper and roast for 10 minutes. Flip the potatoes over and return to the oven for 10 more minutes.

5. Check the potatoes to make sure they are golden brown on the top and bottom. Toss them again, turn the heat down to 350°F, and roast for 30 minutes more.

6. When the potatoes are golden, crispy, and cooked through, sprinkle the Parmesan cheese over them and toss again. Return to the oven for 3 minutes to let the cheese melt a bit.

7. Remove from the oven and sprinkle with the fresh rosemary.

INGREDIENT TIP: If you prefer to use fresh minced garlic instead of powdered, add it with the Parmesan cheese toward the end of the roasting time so it doesn't burn.

Per Serving: Calories: 193; Total fat: 8g; Total carbs: 28g; Fiber: 3g; Sugar: 2g; Protein: 5g; Sodium: 334mg; Cholesterol: 3mg

SPICY WILTED GREENS WITH GARLIC

Prep Time: 10 minutes / Cook Time: 5 minutes / Serves 2
dairy-free, gluten-free, vegan, vegetarian

In the vegetable world, leafy greens reign supreme. They're truly one of the healthiest things you can eat because they're full of so many health-promoting compounds. Eating more greens is linked with better brain health, heart health, and a lower risk of many types of cancer. Cooking them with some olive oil helps to enhance fat-soluble vitamins A, D, E, and K.

1 tablespoon olive oil

2 garlic cloves, minced

3 cups sliced greens (kale, spinach, chard, beet greens, dandelion greens, or a combination)

Pinch salt

Pinch red pepper flakes (or more to taste)

1. Heat the olive oil in a sauté pan over medium-high heat. Add garlic and sauté for 30 seconds, or just until it's fragrant.

2. Add the greens, salt, and pepper flakes and stir to combine. Let the greens wilt, but do not overcook. Remove the pan from the heat and serve.

PREP TIP: I like to cook greens until they're just wilted but still have some crunch. However, if you prefer them softer, reduce the heat and let them cook for another minute or two.

Per Serving: Calories: 91; Total fat: 7g; Total carbs: 7g; Fiber: 3g; Sugar: 1g; Protein: 1g; Sodium: 111mg; Cholesterol: 0mg

ROASTED BROCCOLINI WITH GARLIC AND ROMANO

Prep Time: 5 minutes / Cook Time: 10 minutes / Serves 2
30 minutes, gluten-free, vegetarian

Broccolini, sometimes called baby broccoli, is like broccoli's little cousin. It's a hybrid of broccoli and Chinese broccoli (or gai lan), and it's much quicker cooking and a little bit sweeter than regular broccoli—but every bit as good for you. If you can't find it, you can substitute regular broccoli, but it may need to roast for a bit longer.

1 bunch broccolini (about 5 ounces)

1 tablespoon olive oil

½ teaspoon garlic powder

¼ teaspoon salt

2 tablespoons grated Romano cheese

1. Preheat the oven to 400°F and set the oven rack to the middle position. Line a sheet pan with parchment paper or foil.

2. Slice the tough ends off the broccolini and place in a medium bowl. Add the olive oil, garlic powder, and salt and toss to combine. Arrange broccolini on the lined sheet pan.

3. Roast for 7 minutes, flipping pieces over halfway through the roasting time.

4. Remove the pan from the oven and sprinkle the cheese over the broccolini. With a pair of tongs, carefully flip the pieces over to coat all sides. Return to the oven for another 2 to 3 minutes, or until the cheese melts and starts to turn golden.

PREP TIP: Broccolini cooks fairly quickly and the tops can burn, so if your oven runs hot, you may need to turn it down to 375°F.

SUBSTITUTION TIP: If you don't have Romano cheese on hand, you can substitute grated Parmesan. Keep it in the freezer for longer storage.

Per Serving: Calories: 114; Total fat: 9g; Total carbs: 5g; Fiber: 2g; Sugar: 1g; Protein: 4g; Sodium: 400mg; Cholesterol: 7mg

ROASTED BRUSSELS SPROUTS WITH DELICATA SQUASH AND BALSAMIC GLAZE

Prep Time: 10 minutes / Cook Time: 30 minutes / Serves 2

dairy-free, gluten-free, vegan, vegetarian

Cruciferous vegetables like Brussels sprouts have a bitter flavor, and that's off-putting to many people. However, that bitterness (and the unique smell created when they're cooked) comes from compounds called glucosinolates, which are also responsible for their health benefits. In lab tests, glucosinolates can actually destroy cancer cells, so some bitter is better for you! A note about delicata squash—there's no need to peel it. The skin turns soft when it's roasted and it's perfectly edible. The squash, cranberries, and pomegranate arils are most readily available in the late fall, which makes this a great recipe for the holidays.

½ **pound Brussels sprouts, ends trimmed and outer leaves removed**

1 **medium delicata squash, halved lengthwise, seeded, and cut into 1-inch pieces**

1 **cup fresh cranberries**

2 **teaspoons olive oil**

Salt

Freshly ground black pepper

½ **cup balsamic vinegar**

2 **tablespoons roasted pumpkin seeds**

2 **tablespoons fresh pomegranate arils (seeds)**

1. Preheat oven to 400°F and set the rack to the middle position. Line a sheet pan with parchment paper.

2. Combine the Brussels sprouts, squash, and cranberries in a large bowl. Drizzle with olive oil, and season liberally with salt and pepper. Toss well to coat and arrange in a single layer on the sheet pan.

3. Roast for 30 minutes, turning vegetables halfway through, or until Brussels sprouts turn brown and crisp in spots and squash has golden-brown spots.

4. While vegetables are roasting, prepare the balsamic glaze by simmering the vinegar for 10 to 12 minutes, or until mixture has reduced to about ¼ cup and turns a syrupy consistency.

5. Remove the vegetables from the oven, drizzle with balsamic syrup, and sprinkle with pumpkin seeds and pomegranate arils before serving.

INGREDIENT TIP: When fresh cranberries are in season, grab a few extra bags and store them in the freezer. They'll last for an entire year. Look for pomegranate arils in the prepared foods area of your grocery store produce section.

Per Serving: Calories: 201; Total fat: 7g; Total carbs: 21g; Fiber: 8g; Sugar: 8g; Protein: 6g; Sodium: 34mg; Cholesterol: 0mg

CORIANDER-CUMIN ROASTED CARROTS

Prep Time: 10 minutes / Cook Time: 20 minutes / Serves 2
30 minutes, dairy-free, gluten-free, vegetarian

Carrots are such an easy vegetable to love, especially when they're roasted so their natural sugars caramelize. These hold up very well for leftovers, so double the recipe if you'd like and enjoy them with dinner tomorrow.

½ **pound rainbow carrots (about 4)**

2 tablespoons fresh orange juice

1 tablespoon honey

½ **teaspoon coriander**

Pinch salt

1. Preheat oven to 400°F and set the oven rack to the middle position.

2. Peel the carrots and cut them lengthwise into slices of even thickness. Place them in a large bowl.

3. In a small bowl, mix together the orange juice, honey, coriander, and salt.

4. Pour the orange juice mixture over the carrots and toss well to coat.

5. Spread carrots onto a baking dish in a single layer.

6. Roast for 15 to 20 minutes, or until fork-tender.

SUBSTITUTION TIP: If you can't find rainbow carrots, substitute regular orange carrots or parsnips.

Per Serving: Calories: 85; Total fat: 0g; Total carbs: 21g; Fiber: 3g; Sugar: 16g; Protein: 1g; Sodium: 156mg; Cholesterol: 0mg

GARLIC AND HERB ROASTED GRAPE TOMATOES

Prep Time: 10 minutes / **Cook Time:** 45 minutes / **Serves 2**

dairy-free, gluten-free, vegan, vegetarian

Roasting tomatoes with olive oil helps your body absorb their lycopene content. Lycopene is an important antioxidant that protects your heart, protects your skin from sun damage, and reduces the risk of some types of cancer, especially prostate cancer. Serve these tomatoes as a side, or on top of cooked grains or pasta.

1 pint grape tomatoes

10 whole garlic cloves, skins removed

¼ cup olive oil

½ teaspoon salt

1 fresh rosemary sprig

1 fresh thyme sprig

1. Preheat oven to 350°F.

2. Toss tomatoes, garlic cloves, oil, salt, and herb sprigs in a baking dish.

3. Roast tomatoes until they are soft and begin to caramelize, about 45 minutes.

4. Remove herbs before serving.

PREP TIP: To peel many garlic cloves quickly, place them in a large bowl with a lid or a jar and shake them vigorously. The skins should fall off most of them.

Per Serving: Calories: 271; Total fat: 26g; Total carbs: 12g; Fiber: 3g; Sugar: 5g; Protein: 3g; Sodium: 593mg; Cholesterol: 0mg

ROASTED CAULIFLOWER WITH LEMON TAHINI SAUCE

Prep Time: 10 minutes / Cook Time: 20 minutes / Serves 2

30 minutes, dairy-free, gluten-free, vegan, vegetarian

This recipe not only tastes great; it's also packed with health-promoting ingredients. Cauliflower is a cruciferous vegetable with powerful anticancer properties. Tahini is sesame seed butter, and like all nuts and seeds it's full of heart-healthy, anti-inflammatory fats. Harissa is a Tunisian spice paste full of zesty flavor and antioxidants. When you put them all together, the result is magical.

½ large head cauliflower, stemmed and broken into florets (about 3 cups)

1 tablespoon olive oil

2 tablespoons tahini

2 tablespoons freshly squeezed lemon juice

1 teaspoon harissa paste

Pinch salt

1. Preheat the oven to 400°F and set the rack to the lowest position. Line a sheet pan with parchment paper or foil.

2. Toss the cauliflower florets with the olive oil in a large bowl and transfer to the sheet pan. Reserve the bowl to make the tahini sauce.

3. Roast the cauliflower for 15 minutes, turning it once or twice, until it starts to turn golden.

4. In the same bowl, combine the tahini, lemon juice, harissa, and salt.

5. When the cauliflower is tender, remove it from the oven and toss it with the tahini sauce. Return to the sheet pan and roast for 5 minutes more.

INGREDIENT TIP: Trader Joe's is a good source for harissa paste, but if you can't find it locally you can order it online from spice stores or Amazon. It's a great versatile seasoning to keep on hand.

Per Serving: Calories: 205; Total fat: 15g; Total carbs: 15g; Fiber: 7g; Sugar: 5g; Protein: 7g; Sodium: 161mg; Cholesterol: 0mg

WHITE BEANS WITH ROSEMARY, SAGE, AND GARLIC

Prep Time: 10 minutes / Cook Time: 10 minutes / Serves 2
30 minutes, dairy-free, gluten-free

Beans are honestly the most versatile food: They're perfect in soups, salads, side dishes, and main dishes and can even be used in place of flour and butter in desserts to add moisture and bulk. I love them for their soluble fiber, which lowers cholesterol and blood sugar, and their wide range of nutrients. If there's one food that you really could live on, it would be beans!

1 tablespoon olive oil

2 garlic cloves, minced

1 (15-ounce) can white cannellini beans, drained and rinsed

¼ teaspoon dried sage

1 teaspoon minced fresh rosemary (from 1 sprig) plus 1 whole fresh rosemary sprig

½ cup low-sodium chicken stock

Salt

1. Heat the olive oil in a sauté pan over medium-high heat. Add the garlic and sauté for 30 seconds.

2. Add the beans, sage, minced and whole rosemary, and chicken stock and bring the mixture to a boil.

3. Reduce the heat to medium and simmer the beans for 10 minutes, or until most of the liquid is evaporated. If desired, mash some of the beans with a fork to thicken them.

4. Season with salt. Remove the rosemary sprig before serving

INGREDIENT TIP: Canned beans are one of the best convenience foods to keep on hand. When buying them, look for cans with no salt added so that you can control the amount of sodium in your dish.

Per Serving: Calories: 155; Total fat: 7g; Total carbs: 17g; Fiber: 8g; Sugar: 1g; Protein: 6g; Sodium: 153mg; Cholesterol: 0mg

MOROCCAN-STYLE COUSCOUS

Prep Time: 10 minutes / Cook Time: 5 minutes / Serves 2

30 minutes, dairy-free, vegan, vegetarian

Couscous is the ultimate fast food. It takes just minutes to cook and it serves as a tasty base for stews, meats, beans, or vegetables. This tiny little wheat grain comes from Morocco and North Africa, but it's readily available at all grocery stores. It's a versatile grain that easily adapts to any flavor or cuisine.

1 tablespoon olive oil

¾ cup couscous

¼ teaspoon garlic powder

¼ teaspoon salt

¼ teaspoon cinnamon

1 cup water

2 tablespoons raisins

2 tablespoons minced dried apricots

2 teaspoons minced fresh parsley

1. Heat the olive oil in a saucepan over medium-high heat. Add the couscous, garlic powder, salt, and cinnamon. Stir for 1 minute to toast the couscous and spices.

2. Add the water, raisins, and apricots and bring the mixture to a boil.

3. Cover the pot and turn off the heat. Let the couscous sit for 4 to 5 minutes and then fluff it with a fork. Add parsley and season with additional salt or spices as needed.

INGREDIENT TIP: When buying couscous, make sure you purchase the plain variety instead of the pre-seasoned variety.

Per Serving: Calories: 338; Total fat: 8g; Total carbs: 59g; Fiber: 4g; Sugar: 6g; Protein: 9g; Sodium: 299mg; Cholesterol: 0mg

TOASTED GRAIN AND ALMOND PILAF

Prep Time: 15 minutes / Cook Time: 35 minutes / Serves 2

dairy-free

While you can use any grain here, my personal favorite is barley because it's rich in the kind of fiber that reduces cholesterol. It also has a very low glycemic index compared to other grains, so it helps to stabilize your blood sugar. Toasting it in the pan for a minute before adding liquid gives it a rich, nutty flavor and helps to keep the grains from sticking together.

1 tablespoon olive oil

1 garlic clove, minced

3 scallions, minced

2 ounces mushrooms, sliced

¼ cup sliced almonds

½ cup uncooked pearled barley

1½ cups low-sodium chicken stock

½ teaspoon dried thyme

1 tablespoon fresh minced parsley

Salt

1. Heat the oil in a saucepan over medium-high heat. Add the garlic, scallions, mushrooms, and almonds, and sauté for 3 minutes.

2. Add the barley and cook, stirring, for 1 minute to toast it.

3. Add the chicken stock and thyme and bring the mixture to a boil.

4. Cover and reduce the heat to low. Simmer the barley for 30 minutes, or until the liquid is absorbed and the barley is tender.

5. Sprinkle with fresh parsley and season with salt before serving.

VARIATION TIP: To make this vegan, use water or vegetable stock instead of chicken stock.

Per Serving: Calories: 333; Total fat: 14g; Total carbs: 46g; Fiber: 10g; Sugar: 2g; Protein: 10g; Sodium: 141mg; Cholesterol: 0mg

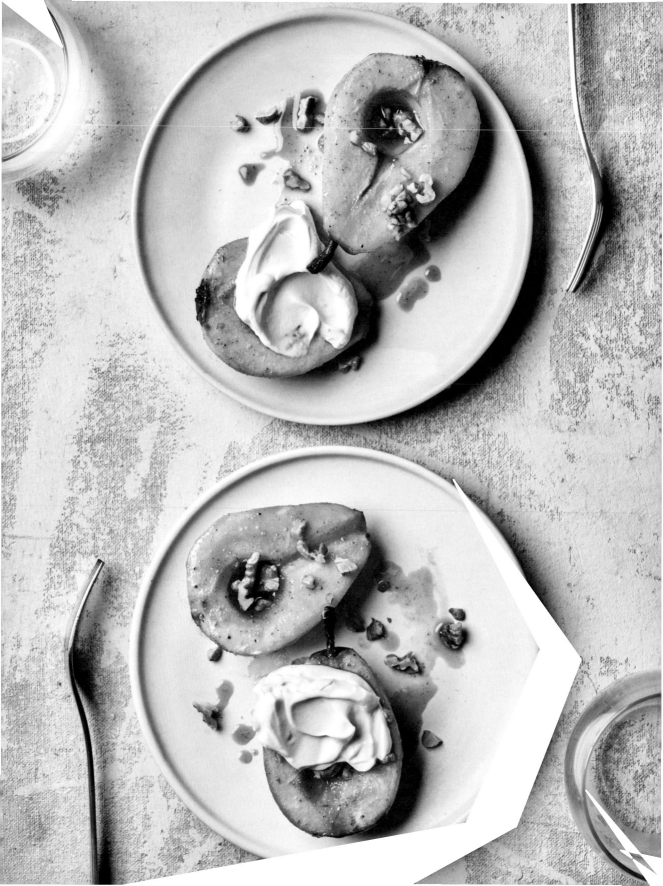

CHAPTER 11

DESSERTS AND SWEETS

Yes, there is room for dessert in the Mediterranean diet! However, sweets and desserts are reserved for holidays and special occasions. You won't find any processed and packaged desserts either. In the Mediterranean diet, desserts are made from whole ingredients, and fruit is usually the star of the dish—or at least a major player.

These desserts do include sugar, but I've tried to limit it, and wherever possible I use honey, maple syrup, or fruit as a sweetener. They still contain sugar, but they have other health benefits that white sugar does not have. Balance is also important, especially when it comes to sweets, so when thinking about dessert I try to balance any sugar or white flour with other nutritious ingredients as much as possible.

< Spiced Baked Pears with Mascarpone, page 166

FLOURLESS CHOCOLATE BROWNIES WITH RASPBERRY BALSAMIC SAUCE

Prep Time: 10 minutes, plus 5 minutes to cool / Cook Time: 20 minutes / Serves 2

dairy-free, gluten-free, vegetarian

The black beans in this skillet brownie are not a typo. They provide moisture and a nice, rich texture, and I promise, if you don't mention them, no one will know they're there. Although this is definitely a sweet treat, the beans also add lots of fiber and protein here, and the dark cocoa powder and raspberry sauce are packed with antioxidants.

For the raspberry sauce

¼ cup good-quality balsamic vinegar

1 cup frozen raspberries

For the brownie

½ cup black beans with no added salt, rinsed

1 large egg

1 tablespoon olive oil

½ teaspoon vanilla extract

4 tablespoons unsweetened cocoa powder

¼ cup sugar

¼ teaspoon baking powder

Pinch salt

¼ cup dark chocolate chips

To make the raspberry sauce

Combine the balsamic vinegar and raspberries in a saucepan and bring the mixture to a boil. Reduce the heat to medium and let the sauce simmer for 15 minutes, or until reduced to ½ cup. If desired, strain the seeds and set the sauce aside until the brownie is ready.

To make the brownie

1. Preheat the oven to 350°F and set the rack to the middle position. Grease two 8-ounce ramekins and place them on a baking sheet.

2. In a food processor, combine the black beans, egg, olive oil, and vanilla. Purée the mixture for 1 to 2 minutes, or until it's smooth and the beans are completely broken down. Scrape down the sides of the bowl a few times to make sure everything is well-incorporated.

3. Add the cocoa powder, sugar, baking powder, and salt and purée again to combine the dry ingredients, scraping down the sides of the bowl as needed.

4. Stir the chocolate chips into the batter by hand. Reserve a few if you like, to sprinkle over the top of the brownies when they come out of the oven.

5. Pour the brownies into the prepared ramekins and bake for 15 minutes, or until firm. The center will look slightly undercooked. If you prefer a firmer brownie, leave it in the oven for another 5 minutes, or until a toothpick inserted in the middle comes out clean.

6. Remove the brownies from the oven. If desired, sprinkle any remaining chocolate chips over the top and let them melt into the warm brownies.

7. Let the brownies cool for a few minutes and top with warm raspberry sauce to serve.

VARIATION TIP: This warm raspberry-balsamic sauce is delicious served over a scoop of vanilla, chocolate, or coconut gelato for a quick no-bake dessert.

Per Serving: Calories: 510; Total fat: 16g; Total carbs: 88g; Fiber: 14g; Sugar: 64g; Protein: 10g; Sodium: 124mg; Cholesterol: 94mg

SPICED BAKED PEARS WITH MASCARPONE

Prep Time: 10 minutes / Cook Time: 20 minutes / Serves 2
30 minutes, gluten-free, vegetarian

Pears are such a treat when they're in season, but sometimes they take a while to ripen, and it's hard to know when they're perfectly ripe. As a result, they tend to get squeezed and bruised too often. The trick is to give them a gentle squeeze on their neck. When the neck yields to gentle pressure, it's ready.

2 ripe pears, peeled

1 tablespoon plus 2 teaspoons honey, divided

1 teaspoon vanilla, divided

¼ teaspoon ginger

¼ teaspoon ground coriander

¼ cup minced walnuts

¼ cup mascarpone cheese

Pinch salt

1. Preheat the oven to 350°F and set the rack to the middle position. Grease a small baking dish.

2. Cut the pears in half lengthwise. Using a spoon, scoop out the core from each piece. Place the pears with the cut side up in the baking dish.

3. Combine 1 tablespoon of honey, ½ teaspoon of vanilla, ginger, and coriander in a small bowl. Pour this mixture evenly over the pear halves.

4. Sprinkle walnuts over the pear halves.

5. Bake for 20 minutes, or until the pears are golden and you're able to pierce them easily with a knife.

6. While the pears are baking, mix the mascarpone cheese with the remaining 2 teaspoons honey, ½ teaspoon of vanilla, and a pinch of salt. Stir well to combine.

7. Divide the mascarpone among the warm pear halves and serve.

SUBSTITUTION TIP: If you don't have ripe pears on hand, try substituting apples. They may need a few more minutes of baking time.

Per Serving: Calories: 307; Total fat: 16g; Total carbs: 43g; Fiber: 6g; Sugar: 31g; Protein: 4g; Sodium: 89mg; Cholesterol: 18mg

ORANGE OLIVE OIL MUG CAKES

Prep Time: 10 minutes / Cook Time: 2 minutes / Serves 2

30 minutes, vegetarian

With just a few ingredients and a cook time of less than two minutes, mug cakes can be a bit dangerous if you have a sweet tooth! The nice thing about them is they satisfy your craving for a piece of cake, and you don't have to worry about portion control. This one is delicious when you have fresh oranges on hand.

6 tablespoons flour

2 tablespoons sugar

½ teaspoon baking powder

Pinch salt

1 teaspoon orange zest

1 egg

2 tablespoons olive oil

2 tablespoons freshly squeezed orange juice

2 tablespoons milk

½ teaspoon orange extract

½ teaspoon vanilla extract

1. In a small bowl, combine the flour, sugar, baking powder, salt, and orange zest.

2. In a separate bowl, whisk together the egg, olive oil, orange juice, milk, orange extract, and vanilla extract.

3. Pour the dry ingredients into the wet ingredients and stir to combine. The batter will be thick.

4. Divide the mixture into two small mugs that hold at least 6 ounces each, or one 12-ounce mug.

5. Microwave each mug separately. The small ones should take about 60 seconds, and one large mug should take about 90 seconds, but microwaves can vary. The cake will be done when it pulls away from the sides of the mug.

VARIATION TIP: To make this dairy-free, substitute a non-dairy milk such as soy, oat, or almond. You can also change up the flavors or add herbs for variety. Try fresh lemon juice with lemon zest and lemon extract and a pinch of lavender buds or fresh lemon thyme.

Per Serving: Calories: 302; Total fat: 17g; Total carbs: 33g; Fiber: 1g; Sugar: 14g; Protein: 6g; Sodium: 117mg; Cholesterol: 83mg

DARK CHOCOLATE BARK WITH FRUIT AND NUTS

Prep Time: 15 minutes, plus 1 hour to cool / Serves 2

dairy-free, gluten-free, vegan, vegetarian

Yes, you can buy dark chocolate bars with fruit and nuts, but the amount of fruit and nuts is often disappointing. It takes just a few minutes to make your own chocolate bark and you can add any type of fruit or nuts you like. I love to make a big batch of this around the holidays. It makes a great hostess gift that's actually much healthier than other sweets.

2 tablespoons chopped nuts (almonds, pecans, walnuts, hazelnuts, pistachios, or any combination of those)

3 ounces good-quality dark chocolate chips (about ⅔ cup)

¼ cup chopped dried fruit (apricots, blueberries, figs, prunes, or any combination of those)

1. Line a sheet pan with parchment paper.

2. Place the nuts in a skillet over medium-high heat and toast them for 60 seconds, or just until they're fragrant.

3. Place the chocolate in a microwave-safe glass bowl or measuring cup and microwave on high for 1 minute. Stir the chocolate and allow any unmelted chips to warm and melt. If necessary, heat for another 20 to 30 seconds, but keep a close eye on it to make sure it doesn't burn.

4. Pour the chocolate onto the sheet pan. Sprinkle the dried fruit and nuts over the chocolate evenly and gently pat in so they stick.

5. Transfer the sheet pan to the refrigerator for at least 1 hour to let the chocolate harden.

6. When solid, break into pieces. Store any leftover chocolate in the refrigerator or freezer.

PREP TIP: Another way to prepare these is to divide the melted chocolate into mini baking cups. Put the cups into a mini muffin pan, fill each with chocolate, and sprinkle the nuts and fruit on top. Use a toothpick to gently push the fruit and nuts into the chocolate.

Per Serving: Calories: 284; Total fat: 16g; Total carbs: 39g; Fiber: 2g; Sugar: 31g; Protein: 4g; Sodium: 2mg; Cholesterol: 0mg

GRILLED FRUIT KEBABS WITH HONEY LABNEH

Prep Time: 15 minutes, plus overnight if making the labneh / Cook Time: 10 minutes / Serves 2

30 minutes, gluten-free, vegetarian

Grilled fruit is a magical treat for your taste buds. When the natural sugars in fruit hit the hot grill, they're intensified and caramelized so much, you'll swear they're soaked in sugar. I love to serve this with honey labneh. Labneh is a Greek yogurt cheese that's carried in some stores, but if you can't find it, it's so easy to make. I use it as a savory spread as in the Herbed Labneh Vegetable Parfaits (page 48), or with a touch of honey as a sweet treat.

⅔ cup prepared labneh, or, if making your own, ⅔ cup full-fat plain Greek yogurt

2 tablespoons honey

1 teaspoon vanilla extract

Pinch salt

3 cups fresh fruit cut into 2-inch chunks (pineapple, cantaloupe, nectarines, strawberries, plums, or mango)

1. If making your own labneh, place a colander over a bowl and line it with cheesecloth. Place the Greek yogurt in the cheesecloth and wrap it up. Put the bowl in the refrigerator and let sit for at least 12 to 24 hours, until it's thick like soft cheese.

2. Mix honey, vanilla, and salt into labneh. Stir well to combine and set it aside.

3. Heat the grill to medium (about 300°F) and oil the grill grate. Alternatively, you can cook these on the stovetop in a heavy grill pan (cast iron works well).

4. Thread the fruit onto skewers and grill for 4 minutes on each side, or until fruit is softened and has grill marks on each side.

5. Serve the fruit with labneh to dip.

Per Serving: Calories: 292; Total fat: 6g; Total carbs: 60g; Fiber: 4g; Sugar: 56g; Protein: 5g; Sodium: 131mg; Cholesterol: 17mg

BLUEBERRY POMEGRANATE GRANITA

Prep Time: 5 minutes / Cook Time: 10 minutes, plus 30 minutes to cool and
2 hours to freeze / Serves 2

dairy-free, gluten-free, vegan, vegetarian

A granita is a refreshing frozen fruit ice, the more grown-up version of a snow cone. Wild blueberries, which are almost always sold frozen, have a sweeter flavor and are higher in antioxidants than the larger blueberries in the produce department.

1 cup frozen
wild blueberries

1 cup pomegranate
or pomegranate
blueberry juice

¼ cup sugar

¼ cup water

1. Combine the frozen blueberries and pomegranate juice in a saucepan and bring to a boil. Reduce the heat and simmer for 5 minutes, or until the blueberries start to break down.

2. While the juice and berries are cooking, combine the sugar and water in a small microwave-safe bowl. Microwave for 60 seconds, or until it comes to a rolling boil. Stir to make sure all of the sugar is dissolved and set the syrup aside.

3. Combine the blueberry mixture and the sugar syrup in a blender and blend for 1 minute, or until the fruit is completely puréed.

4. Pour the mixture into an 8-by-8-inch baking pan or a similar-sized bowl. The liquid should come about ½ inch up the sides. Let the mixture cool for 30 minutes, and then put it into the freezer.

5. Every 30 minutes for the next 2 hours, scrape the granita with a fork to keep it from freezing solid.

6. Serve it after 2 hours, or store it in a covered container in the freezer.

Per Serving: Calories: 214; Total fat: 0g; Total carbs: 54g; Fiber: 2g; Sugar: 48g; Protein: 1g; Sodium: 15mg; Cholesterol: 0mg

MINI MIXED BERRY CRUMBLES

Prep Time: 15 minutes / Cook Time: 30 minutes / Serves 2

gluten-free, vegan, vegetarian

Frozen fruit is technically a processed food, but it's one that I recommend keeping stocked in your freezer—just make sure there's no sugar added. The best thing about frozen fruit is that it keeps for months, so you can use small amounts for a recipe like this. Mixed berries are one of my favorites. They're high in healthy antioxidants, and they have a low glycemic index, so they won't raise your blood sugar very quickly. Berries are also linked to heart and brain health.

1½ cups frozen mixed berries, thawed

1 tablespoon butter, softened

1 tablespoon brown sugar

¼ cup pecans

¼ cup oats

1. Preheat the oven to 350°F and set the rack to the middle position.

2. Divide the berries between 2 (8-ounce) ramekins

3. In a food processor, combine the butter, brown sugar, pecans, and oats, and pulse a few times, until the mixture resembles damp sand.

4. Divide the crumble topping over the berries.

5. Place the ramekins on a sheet pan and bake for 30 minutes, or until the top is golden and the berries are bubbling.

INGREDIENT TIP: When buying frozen berries, look for organic. Berries can be a high-pesticide fruit, and while fresh organic berries can be expensive, often the frozen ones are a more reasonable price.

Per Serving: Calories: 267; Total fat: 17g; Total carbs: 27g; Fiber: 6g; Sugar: 13g; Protein: 4g; Sodium: 43mg; Cholesterol: 15mg

CHOCOLATE TURTLE HUMMUS

Prep Time: 15 minutes / Serves 2

30 minutes, dairy-free, gluten-free, vegan, vegetarian

Hummus and chocolate might not sound like they go together, but please keep an open mind on this, because it's amazing. I've been making dessert hummus for a while, and now I'm seeing it pop up in grocery stores, so it really is a thing! This chocolate turtle flavor is my favorite dessert flavor hummus so far. It tastes like chocolate turtle candy, but it's made from only wholesome ingredients, and it's packed with fiber and protein from chickpeas.

For the caramel

2 tablespoons coconut oil

1 tablespoon maple syrup

1 tablespoon almond butter

Pinch salt

For the hummus

½ cup chickpeas, drained and rinsed

2 tablespoons unsweetened cocoa powder

1 tablespoon maple syrup, plus more to taste

2 tablespoons almond milk, or more as needed, to thin

Pinch salt

2 tablespoons pecans

To make the caramel

1. To make the caramel, put the coconut oil in a small microwave-safe bowl. If it's solid, microwave it for about 15 seconds to melt it.

2. Stir in the maple syrup, almond butter, and salt.

3. Place the caramel in the refrigerator for 5 to 10 minutes to thicken.

To make the hummus

1. In a food processor, combine the chickpeas, cocoa powder, maple syrup, almond milk, and pinch of salt, and process until smooth. Scrape down the sides to make sure everything is incorporated.

2. If the hummus seems too thick, add another table-spoon of almond milk.

3. Add the pecans and pulse 6 times to roughly chop them.

4. Transfer the hummus to a serving bowl and when the caramel is thickened, swirl it into the hummus. Gently fold it in, but don't mix it in completely.

5. Serve with fresh fruit or pretzels.

PREP TIP: Chickpeas often have loose skins on them. If the texture bothers you, put the rinsed chickpeas in a large bowl of water, rub them with your fingers, and let the skins float to the top so you can strain them off.

Per Serving: Calories: 321; Total fat: 22g; Total carbs: 30g; Fiber: 6g; Sugar: 15g; Protein: 7g; Sodium: 100mg; Cholesterol: 0mg

LEMON PANNA COTTA WITH BLACKBERRIES

Prep Time: 20 minutes / Cook Time: 10 minutes, plus 6 hours to set / Serves 2

30 minutes, gluten-free, vegetarian

Panna cotta is Italian for "cooked cream," and it's a simple but luscious dessert that's perfect for a special occasion. The heavy cream makes this dish very rich, so a small portion topped with some fresh berries is all you need. I love the lemon flavor with blackberries, but raspberries or fresh blueberries would be lovely too.

¾ **cup half-and-half, divided**

1 **teaspoon unflavored powdered gelatin**

½ **cup heavy cream**

3 **tablespoons sugar**

1 **teaspoon lemon zest**

1 **tablespoon freshly squeezed lemon juice**

1 **teaspoon lemon extract**

½ **cup fresh blackberries**

Lemon peels to garnish (optional)

1. Place ¼ cup of half-and-half in a small bowl.

2. Sprinkle the gelatin powder evenly over the half-and-half and set it aside for 10 minutes to hydrate.

3. In a saucepan, combine the remaining ½ cup of half-and-half, the heavy cream, sugar, lemon zest, lemon juice, and lemon extract. Heat the mixture over medium heat for 4 minutes, or until it's barely simmering—don't let it come to a full boil. Remove from the heat.

4. When the gelatin is hydrated (it will look like applesauce), add it into the warm cream mixture, whisking as the gelatin melts.

5. If there are any remaining clumps of gelatin, strain the liquid or remove the lumps with a spoon.

6. Pour the mixture into 2 dessert glasses or stemless wineglasses and refrigerate for at least 6 hours, or up to overnight.

7. Serve with the fresh berries and garnish with some strips of fresh lemon peel, if desired.

PREP TIP: Gelatin doesn't dissolve as well in hot liquid, so make sure you hydrate it (also called "blooming") in cold liquid first.

Per Serving: Calories: 422; Total fat: 33g; Total carbs: 28g; Fiber: 2g; Sugar: 21g; Protein: 6g; Sodium: 64mg; Cholesterol: 115mg

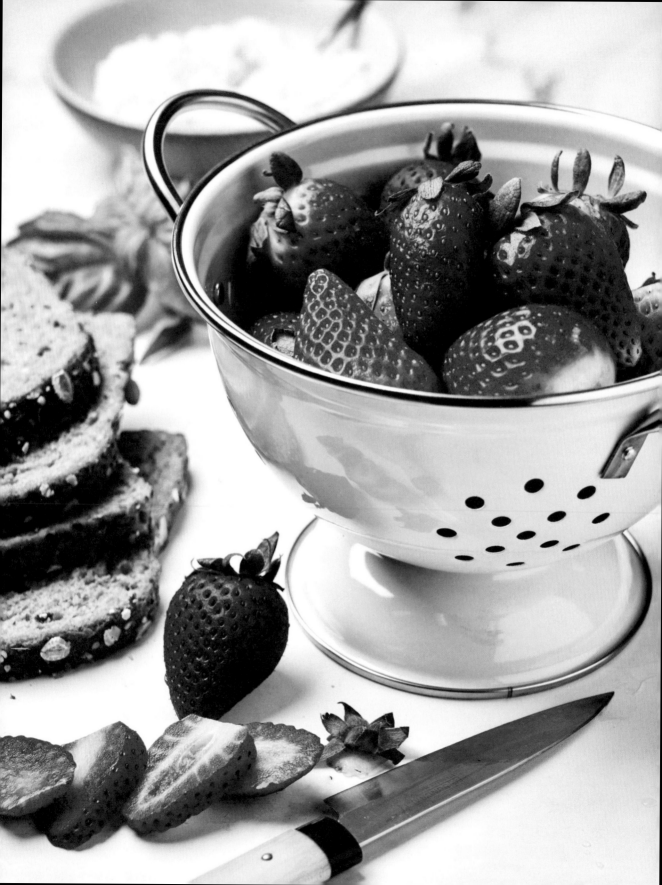

MEASUREMENT CONVERSIONS

VOLUME EQUIVALENTS (LIQUID)

STANDARD	US STANDARD (OUNCES)	METRIC (APPROXIMATE)
2 tablespoons	1 fl. oz.	30 mL
¼ cup	2 fl. oz.	60 mL
½ cup	4 fl. oz.	120 mL
1 cup	8 fl. oz.	240 mL
1½ cups	12 fl. oz.	355 mL
2 cups or 1 pint	16 fl. oz.	475 mL
4 cups or 1 quart	32 fl. oz.	1 L
1 gallon	128 fl. oz.	4 L

OVEN TEMPERATURES

FAHRENHEIT (F)	CELSIUS (C) (APPROXIMATE)
250°	120°
300°	150°
325°	165°
350°	180°
375°	190°
400°	200°
425°	220°
450°	230°

VOLUME EQUIVALENTS (DRY)

STANDARD	METRIC (APPROXIMATE)
⅛ teaspoon	0.5 mL
¼ teaspoon	1 mL
½ teaspoon	2 mL
¾ teaspoon	4 mL
1 teaspoon	5 mL
1 tablespoon	15 mL
¼ cup	59 mL
⅓ cup	79 mL
½ cup	118 mL
⅔ cup	156 mL
¾ cup	177 mL
1 cup	235 mL
2 cups or 1 pint	475 mL
3 cups	700 mL
4 cups or 1 quart	1 L

WEIGHT EQUIVALENTS

STANDARD	METRIC (APPROXIMATE)
½ ounce	15 g
1 ounce	30 g
2 ounces	60 g
4 ounces	115 g
8 ounces	225 g
12 ounces	340 g
16 ounces or 1 pound	455 g

REFERENCES

Alonso-Molero, Jessica, Carmen González-Donquiles, Camillo Palazuelos, Tania Fernández-Villa, Elena Ramos, Marina Pollán, Nuria Aragonés, Javier Llorca, M. Henar Alonso, Adonina Tardón, et al. "The RS4939827 Polymorphism in the SMAD7 GENE and Its Association with Mediterranean Diet in Colorectal Carcinogenesis." *BMC Medical Genetics* 18, no. 1 (October 2017): 122.

Altomare, Roberta, Francesco Cacciabaudo, Giuseppe Damiano, Vincenzo Davide Palumbo, Maria Concetta Gioviale, Maurizio Bellavia, Giovanni Tomasello, and Attilio Ignacio Lo Monte. "The Mediterranean Diet: A History of Health." *Iran Journal of Public Health* 42, no. 5 (May 2013): 449–57. https://www.ncbi.nlm.nih.gov/pmc/articles/PMC3684452.

Amati, Federica, Sondus Hassounah, and Alexandra Swaka. "The Impact of Mediterranean Dietary Patterns During Pregnancy on Maternal and Offspring Health." *Nutrients* 11, no. 5 (May 2019): 1098.

Ascherio, Alberto, and Walter C. Willett. "Health Effects of Trans Fatty Acids." *American Journal of Clinical Nutrition* 66, no. 4 (October 1997): 1006S–10S. https://www.ncbi.nlm.nih.gov/pubmed/9322581.

Babio, Nancy, Estefanía Toledo, Ramon Estruch, Emilio Ros, Miguel Ángel Martínez-González, Olga Castañer, Monica Bulló, Dolores Corella, Fernando Arós, Enrique Gómez-Gracia, et al. "Mediterranean Diets and Metabolic Syndrome Status in the PREDIMED Randomized Trial." *Canadian Medical Association Journal* 186, no. 17 (November 2014): E649–57.

Basterra-Gortari, F. Javier, Miguel Ruiz-Canela, Miguel A. Martínez-González, Nancy Babio, José V. Sorlí, Montserrat Fito, Emilio Ros, Enrique Gómez-Gracia, Miquel Fiol, José Lapetra, et al. "Effects of a Mediterranean Eating Plan on the Need for Glucose-Lowering Medications in Participants With Type 2 Diabetes: A Subgroup Analysis of the PREDIMED Trial." *Diabetes Care* 42, no. 8 (August 2019): 1390–97.

Castelló, Adela, Elena Boldo, Pilar Amiano, Gemma Castaño-Vinyals, Nuria Aragonés, Inés Gómez-Acebo, Rosana Peiró, Jose Juan Jimenez-Moleón, Juan Alguacil, Adonina Tardón, et al. "Mediterranean Dietary Pattern Is Associated with Low Risk of Aggressive Prostate Cancer: MCC-Spain Study." *Journal of Urology* 199, no. 2 (February 2018): 430–7.

Choi, Eunhee, Seong-Ah Kim, and Hyojee Joung. "Relationship between Obesity and Korean and Mediterranean Dietary Patterns: A Review of the Literature." *Journal of Obesity and Metabolic Syndrome* 28, no. 1 (2019): 30–39. doi:10.7570/jomes.2019.28.1.30.

Davis, Courtney, Janet Bryan, Jonathan Hodgson, and Karen Murphy. "Definition of the Mediterranean Diet; a Literature Review." *Nutrients* 7, no. 11 (November 2015): 9139–53. https://doi.org/10.3390/nu7115459.

de Lorgeril Michel, Patricia Salen, Jean-Louis Martin, Isabelle Monjaud, Jacques Delaye, and Nicole Mamelle. "Mediterranean Diet, Traditional Risk Factors, and the Rate of Cardiovascular Complications after Myocardial Infarction: Final Report of the Lyon Diet Heart Study." *Circulation* 99, no. 6 (February 1999): 779–85. https://doi.org/10.1161/01.CIR.99.6.779.

de Souza Russell J., Andrew Mente, Adriana Maroleanu, Adrian I. Cozma, Vanessa Ha, Teruko Kishibe, Elizabeth Uleryk, Patrick Budylowski, Holger Schünemann, Joseph Beyene, et al. "Intake of Saturated and Trans Unsaturated Fatty Acids and Risk of All Cause Mortality, Cardiovascular Disease, and Type 2 Diabetes: Systematic Review and Meta-Analysis of Observational Studies. *BMJ* 351 (August 2015): h3978. https://www.ncbi.nlm.nih.gov/pmc/articles /PMC4532752.

Estruch, Ramon, Miguel Ángel Martínez-González, Dolores Corella, Jordi Salas-Salvadó, Montserrat Fitó, Gemma Chiva-Blanch, Miquel Fiol, Enrique Gómez-Gracia, Fernando Arós, José Lapetra, et al. "Effect of a High-Fat Mediterranean Diet on Bodyweight and Waist Circumference: A Prespecified Secondary Outcomes Analysis of the PREDIMED Randomised Controlled Trial." *Lancet Diabetes & Endocrinology* 4, no. 8 (August 2016): 666–76.

Estruch, Ramon, Emilio Ros, Jordi Salas-Salvadó, Maria-Isabel Covas, Dolores Corella, Fernando Arós, Enrique Gómez-Gracia, Valenina Ruiz-Gutiérrez, Miquel Fiol, et al. "Primary Prevention of Cardiovascular Disease with a Mediterranean Diet Supplemented with Extra-Virgin Olive Oil or Nuts." *New England Journal of Medicine* 378, no. 25 (June 2018): e34. https://www.ncbi.nlm.nih.gov/pubmed/29897866.

Filomeno, Maria, Cristina Bosetti, E. Bidoli, F. Levi, Diego Serraino, Maurizio Montella, C. La Vecchia, and A. Tavani. "Mediterranean Diet and Risk of Endometrial Cancer: A Pooled Analysis of Three Italian Case-Control Studies." *British Journal of Cancer* 112, no. 11 (May 2015): 1816.

Franquesa, Marcella, Georgina Pujol-Busquets Guillen, Elena García-Fernández, Laura Rico, Laia Shamirian-Pulido, Alicia Aguilar-Martínez, Francesc Xavier Medina, Lluis Serra-Majem, and Anna Bach-Faig. "Mediterranean Diet and Cardiodiabesity: A Systematic Review through Evidence-Based Answers to Key Clinical Questions." *Nutrients* 11, no. 3 (March 2019): 655.

Fung, Teresa T., Katherine M. Rexrode, Christos S. Mantzoros, JoAnn E. Manson, Walter C. Willett, and Frank B. Hu. "Mediterranean Diet and Incidence and Mortality of Coronary Heart Disease and Stroke in Women." *Circulation* 119, no. 8 (March 2009): 1093. https://www.ncbi.nlm.nih.gov/pmc/articles/PMC2724471.

Georgousopoulou, Ekavi N., Christos Pitsavos, Demosthenes Panagiotakos, Christine Chrysohoou, et al. "Adherence to Mediterranean Is the Most Important Protector Against the Development of Fatal and Non-Fatal Cardiovascular Event: 10-year Follow-up (2002–12) of the Attica Study." *Journal of the American College of Cardiology* 65, no. 10 Supplement (March 2015): A1449.

Hernáez, Álvaro, Olga Castañer, Roberto Elosua, Xavier Pintó X, Ramon Estruch, Jordi Salas-Salvadó, Dolores Corella, Fernando Arós, Lluis Serra-Majem, Miquel Fiol, et al. "Mediterranean Diet Improves High-Density Lipoprotein Function in High-Cardiovascular-Risk Individuals: A Randomized Controlled Trial." *Circulation* 135, no.7 (February 2017): 633–43.

Hoşcan, Yeşim, Fatma Yiğit, and Haldun Müderrisoğlu. "Adherence to Mediterranean Diet and Its Relation with Cardiovascular Diseases in Turkish Population." *International Journal of Clinical and Experimental Medicine* 8, no. 2 (2015): 2860.

Kastorini, Christina-Maria, Haralampos J. Milionis, Katherine Esposito, Dario Giugliano, John A. Goudevenos, and Demosthenes B. Panagiotakos. "The Effect of Mediterranean Diet on Metabolic Syndrome and Its Components: A Meta-Analysis of 50 studies and 534,906 Individuals." *Journal of the American College of Cardiology* 57, no. 11 (March 2011): 1299–313.

Klonizakis, Markos, Ahmad Alkhatib, and Geoff Middleton. "Long-Term Effects of an Exercise and Mediterranean Diet Intervention in the Vascular Function of an Older, Healthy Population." *Microvascular Research* 95 (September 2014): 103–7.

Lassale, Camille, G. David Batty, Amaria Baghdadli, Felicia Jacka, Almudena Sánchez-Villegas, Mika Kivimäki, and Tasnime Akbaraly. "Healthy Dietary Indices and Risk of Depressive Outcomes: A Systematic Review and Meta-Analysis of Observational Studies." *Molecular Psychiatry* 24, no. 7 (July 2019): 965–86.

Mattioli, Anna V., F. Coppi, Mario Migaldi, Pietro Scicchitano, Marco M. Ciccone, Alberto Farinetti. "Relationship Between Mediterranean Diet and Asymptomatic Peripheral Arterial Disease in a Population of Pre-Menopausal Women." *Nutrition, Metabolism and Cardiovascular Diseases* 27, no. 11 (November 2018): 985–90.

McEvoy, Claire T., Tina Hoang, Stephen Sidney, Lyn M. Steffen, David R. Jacobs, James M. Shikany, John T. Wilkins, and Kristine Yaffe. "Dietary Patterns during Adulthood and Cognitive Performance in Midlife: The CARDIA Study." *Neurology* 92, no. 14 (April 2019): e1589–99.

Oldways. "Mediterranean Diet." Accessed October 27, 2019. https://oldwayspt .org/traditional-diets/mediterranean-diet.

The Online Scientist. "Study Findings." The Seven Countries Study. https://www .sevencountriesstudy.com/study-findings.

Rainey-Smith, Stephanie R., Yian Gu, Samantha L. Gardener, James D. Doecke, Victor L. Villemagne, Belinda M. Brown, Kevin Taddei, Simon M. Laws, Hamid R. Sohrabi, Michael Weinborn, et al. "Mediterranean Diet Adherence and Rate of Cerebral Aß-amyloid Accumulation: Data from the Australian Imaging, Biomarkers and Lifestyle Study of Ageing." *Translational Psychiatry* 8, no. 1 (October 2018): 238.

Richard, Caroline, Patrick Couture, Sophie Desroches, Suzanne Benjannet, Nabil G. Seidah, Alice H. Lichtenstein, and Benoit Lamarche. "Effect of the Mediterranean Diet with and without Weight Loss on Surrogate Markers of Cholesterol Homeostasis in Men with the Metabolic Syndrome." *British Journal of Nutrition* 107, no. 5 (March 2012): 705–11.

Salas-Salvadó, Jordi, Monica Bulló, Nancy Babio, Miguel Ángel Martínez-González, Núria Ibarrola-Jurado, Josep Basora, Ramon Estruch, Maria Isabel Covas, Dolores Corella, Fernando Arós, et al. "Reduction in the Incidence of Type 2 Diabetes with the Mediterranean Diet: Results of the PREDIMED-Reus Nutrition Intervention Randomized Trial." *Diabetes Care* 34, no. 1 (January): 14. https://www.ncbi.nlm.nih.gov/pmc/articles/PMC3005482.

Schwingshackl, Lulas, Anna-Maria Lampousi, M. P. Portillo, D. Romaguera, Georg Hoffmann, and H. Boeing. "Olive Oil in the Prevention and Management of Type 2 Diabetes Mellitus: A Systematic Review and Meta-Analysis of Cohort Studies and Intervention Trials." *Nutrition & Diabetes* 7, no. 4 (April 2017): e262.

Vallance, Jeff K., Paul A. Gardiner, Brigid M. Lynch, Adrijana D'Silva, Terry Boyle, Lorian M. Taylor, Stephen T. Johnson, Matthew P. Buman, and Neville Owen. "Evaluating the Evidence on Sitting, Smoking, and Health: Is Sitting Really the New Smoking?" *American Journal of Public Health* 108, no. 11 (November 2018): 1478–82.

van den Brandt, Piet A., and Maya Schulpen. "Mediterranean Diet Adherence and Risk of Postmenopausal Breast Cancer: Results of a Cohort Study and Meta-Analysis." *International Journal of Cancer* 140, no. 10 (May 2017): 2220-31.

Violi, Franceso, Lorenzo Loffredo, Pasquale Pignatelli, Francesco Angelico, Simona Bartimoccia, Cristina Nocella, Roberto Cangemi, Andreina Petruccioli, Roberto Monticolo, Daniele Pastori, et al. "Extra Virgin Olive Oil Use is Associated with Improved Post-Prandial Blood Glucose and LDL cholesterol in Healthy Subjects." *Nutrition & Diabetes* 5, no. 7 (July 2015): e172.

Wade, Alexandra T., Merrill F. Elias, and Karen J. Murphy. "Adherence to a Mediterranean Diet is Associated with Cognitive Function in an Older Non-Mediterranean Sample: Findings from the Maine-Syracuse Longitudinal Study." *Nutritional Neuroscience* (August 2019): 1–2.

Witlox, Willem J. A., Fritz H. M. van Osch, Maree Brinkman, Sylvia Jochems, Maria E. Goossens, Elisabete Weiderpass, Emily White, Piet A. van den Brandt, Graham G. Giles, Roger L. Milne, et al. "An Inverse Association Between the Mediterranean Diet and Bladder Cancer Risk: A Pooled Analysis of 13 Cohort Studies." *European Journal of Nutrition* (February 2019): 1–10.

INDEX

ABOUT THE AUTHOR

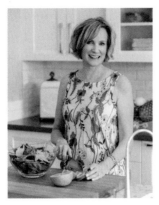 **Anne Danahy, RDN,** is a registered dietitian and free-lance health and nutrition writer who specializes in integrative nutrition, disease prevention, and healthy aging. She believes living well begins with eating well, and as such, she promotes a balanced diet of foods low on the glycemic index, lots of plants, and everything in moderation sprinkled in.

With over 25 years of nutrition and communications experience, Anne works with individuals and groups, as well as brands, food commodities, and the media to inspire her audience to eat better, age gracefully, and live vibrantly. This is her first cookbook.

Anne blogs at CravingSomethingHealthy.com, where she enjoys helping others make sense of the latest nutrition research and get it onto their plates in the most delicious way possible.